Cancer Drug Discovery and Development

Series Editor: Beverly A. Teicher

For other titles published in this series, go to
http://www.springer.com/series/7625

Amy M. Fulton
Editor

Chemokine Receptors in Cancer

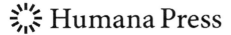 Humana Press

Editor

Amy M. Fulton
Department of Pathology
School of Medicine
Marlene and Stewart
 Greenebaum Cancer Center
University of Maryland
Baltimore MD 21201
USA
afulton@umaryland.edu

ISBN 978-1-60327-266-7   e-ISBN 978-1-60327-267-4
DOI 10.1007/978-1-60327-267-4

Library of Congress Control Number: 2009921125

springer.com

Preface

The chemokine receptors are a diverse family of seven-transmembrane G-protein-coupled receptors binding a large family of ligands. Chemokine receptors were first identified on leukocytes and mediate directed migration of many host cells to sites of ligand expression. It is now well established that most malignant cells also express one or more chemokine receptor. This volume will summarize the growing body of evidence that several chemokine receptors contribute to tumor behavior.

There is abundant evidence that CXCR4, which is widely expressed in many malignancies, contributes to the ability of tumor cells to metastasize to sites of ligand expression. Evidence for regulation of CXCR4 by hypoxia is described. Like CXCR4, both CCR7 and CXCR3 function to promote tumor cell homing and metastasis of melanoma, breast and colon cancers. Several chemokine receptors also function to support the survival and proliferation of tumor cells either directly or through transactivation by tyrosine kinase-coupled growth factor receptors.

While chemokine receptors expressed on tumor cells generally support tumor growth and dissemination, expression of these receptors on host cells has both pro-tumor and anti-tumor functions. Both angiostatic and angiogeneic functions of CXC chemokines acting on endothelial cells have been described. The CXCR3 receptor expressed on malignant cells promotes metastasis but CXCR3+ Th1 cells and NK cells play a protective role in several tumor models. Data demonstrating the potential therapeutic potential of CXCR3 ligand overexpression acting on host immune and endothelial cells are also summarized. The CCR5/CCL5 axis has a complex role in tumor behavior with induction of an early protective T-cell response that is ultimately overridden by a tumor growth-promoting role of CCL5.

There are also several chemokine receptors that act as decoy receptors, binding ligands with high affinity. Although these receptors do not transduce signals that mediate intracellular responses, ligand binding does contribute to tumor behavior. For example, the D6 receptor may act as a biological sink to reduce the bioavailability of pro-angiogenic chemokines. Differences in decoy receptor expression in different populations may contribute to disparities in cancer incidence and outcome.

The therapeutic potential and challenges of targeting chemokine receptors in cancer is also discussed. Based on promising preclinical data, antagonists of CXCR4 are currently being evaluated in clinical trials. Initial studies have indicated that inhibition of several other chemokine receptors, expressed on the malignant cell, shows promise; however, this approach is complicated by the fact that many protective host cells express the same receptors. In summary, the study of chemokine receptors in cancer has rapidly expanded since the initial description, in 2001, of CXCR4 and CCR7 in cancer cells. Many studies attest to the importance of chemokine receptors as determinants of tumor behavior. The current challenge is to understand the mechanisms underlying these functions and to more effectively target these receptors therapeutically.

Amy M. Fulton
Baltimore, MD, USA

Contents

Contributors

Chareeporn Akekawatchai Chemokine Biology Laboratory, The School of Molecular and Biomedical Science, The University of Adelaide, Adelaide, SA 5005, Australia

Adit Ben-Baruch Department of Cell Research and Immunology, George S. Wise Faculty of Life Sciences, Tel Aviv University, Tel Aviv 69978, Israel

Thorsten Eismann Department of Surgery, University of Cincinnati College of Medicine, Cincinnati, OH 45267-0558, USA

Lei Fang Dermatology Branch, National Cancer Institute, Center for Cancer Research, Bethesda, MD 20892, USA

Amy M. Fulton Marlene and Stewart Greenebaum Cancer Center and Department of Pathology, University of Maryland School of Medicine, 655 West Baltimore Street, Baltimore MD 21201, USA

Bungo Furusato Center for Prostate Disease Research, Department of Surgery, Uniformed Service University of the Health Science, Bethesda, MD 20814; Department of Genitourinary Pathology, Armed Forces Institute of Pathology Washington, DC 20307, USA

Jane Holland Chemokine Biology Laboratory, The School of Molecular and Biomedical Science, North Terrace Campus, Level 5, The University of Adelaide, Adelaide, SA 5005, Australia

Nadine Huber Department of Surgery, University of Cincinnati College of Medicine, Cincinnati, OH 45267-0558, USA

Sam T. Hwang Department of Dermatology, Medical College of Wisconsin, Milwaukee, WI 53226, USA

Kenji Kawada Department of Surgery, Graduate School of Medicine, Kyoto University, Sakyo, Kyoto 606-8501, Japan

Marina Kochetkova Chemokine Biology Laboratory, The School of Molecular and Biomedical Science, The University of Adelaide, Adelaide, SA 5005, Australia

Alex B. Lentsch Department of Surgery, University of Cincinnati College of Medicine, Cincinnati, OH 45267-0558, USA

Yanchun Li Marlene and Stewart Greenebaum Cancer Center, University of Maryland School of Medicine, Baltimore, MD 21201, USA

Shaun R. McColl Chemokine Biology Laboratory, The School of Molecular and Biomedical Science, The University of Adelaide, South Australia, 5005

Borna Mehrad Division of Pulmonary and Critical Care Medicine, Department of Medicine, University of Virginia, Charlottesville, VA 22908, USA

Elizabeth W. Newcomb Department of Pathology, New York University Cancer Institute, New York University School of Medicine, New York, NY 10016, USA

Johng S. Rhim Department of Surgery, Center for Prostate Disease Research, Uniformed Service University of the Health Science, Bethesda, MD 20814, USA

Gali Soria Department Cell Research and Immunology, George S. Wise Faculty of Life Sciences, Tel Aviv University, Tel Aviv 69978, Israel

Robert M. Strieter Division of Pulmonary and Critical Care Medicine, Department of Medicine, University of Virginia, Charlottesville, VA 22908, USA

Makoto Mark Taketo Department of Pharmacology, Graduate School of Medicine, Kyoto University, Sakyo, Kyoto 606-8501, Japan

David Zagzag Department of Pathology and Division of Neuropathology and Department of Neurosurgery, New York University Cancer Institute, New York University School of Medicine, New York, NY 10016, USA

Chemokines and Chemokine Receptors in Cancer Progression

Chareeporn Akekawatchai, Marina Kochetkova, Jane Holland, and Shaun R. McColl

Abstract Directed cell migration is a fundamental component of numerous biological systems and is critical to the pathology of many diseases. Although the importance of chemokines in providing navigational cues to migrating cells bearing specific receptors is well-established, how chemokine function is regulated is not so well understood and may be of key importance to the design of new therapeutics for numerous human diseases, particularly for the control of cancer growth and metastasis, diseases in which chemokines have recently been implicated. In this review, we discuss the general views on the role of specific chemokines in these pathological processes. In addition, we discuss two novel aspects of chemokine cancer biology; cross-talk between chemokine and growth factor receptors, and refractory chemokine receptors.

Introduction

Cancer comprises a large group of diseases which share an important characteristic of uncontrolled growth. In most tissues and organs, homeostasis is maintained by a balance between cell proliferation and cell death. Occasionally, cells lose the ability to respond to the normal growth control mechanisms and clones of cells arise which can expand to a considerable size producing tumours or neoplasms. A tumour that remains in its original location, is not able to grow indefinitely and does not invade surrounding tissue is termed benign, whereas a tumour which grows extensively and becomes invasive is known as a malignant tumour or cancer. In addition, most malignant tumours are able to metastasize, a process of new tumour formation and growth in distant organs, which is the cause of 90% of human deaths from cancer [115].

Studies on the molecular biology of tumour progression have emphasized the importance of the interaction between the tumour and host homeostatic

C. Akekawatchai (✉)
Chemokine Biology Laboratory, The School of Molecular and Biomedical Science,
The University of Adelaide, Adelaide, SA 5005, Australia

A.M. Fulton (ed.), *Chemokine Receptors in Cancer*, Cancer Drug Discovery and Development, DOI 10.1007/978-1-60327-267-4_1,
© Humana Press, a part of Springer Science+Business Media, LLC 2009

systems. Accumulating data support the roles of various types of host cells, such as immune cells, endothelial cells, fibroblasts and platelets, and their cytokines, particularly in the establishment of the tumour microenvironment [58, 106]. At the tumour–host interface, a wide range of host factors including growth factors, adhesion molecules, cytokines and chemoattractants support tumour cell proliferation, survival and migration that promote growth and invasion of tumours [82]. Recently, members of chemoattractant cytokines, named chemokines, which were primarily known as key regulators of the immune system, have been implicated in many facets of malignant transformation and tumour progression [7, 49, 121, 129]. Most importantly, a growing body of experimental evidence both *in vitro* and *in vivo* suggests that members of the chemokine family together with their cognate receptors play a key role in the metastatic progression of numerous tumour types [49]. Various functions and modes of action have been proposed for chemokines and their receptors in the development of primary and secondary tumours, which together with the underlying genetic and molecular mechanisms are extensively covered in the recent scientific literature. This chapter will focus on the current advances in the understanding of the role of the chemokine receptor family of proteins in the progression of tumours to malignancy. Also, the recently discovered novel aspects in the pathobiology of chemokine receptors that are specifically associated with the invasive phenotype of cancer cells will be discussed.

Tumourigenesis, Invasion and Metastasis

Tumour progression to invasion and metastasis is a complex process that consists of sequential and interrelated steps [22, 35, 36]. When cellular transformation occurs at the primary site, the growth of a neoplasm is supported initially by simple diffusion of nutrients in an expanding tumour mass; however, vascularization must initiate if a tumour mass is to exceed $1–2\,mm^3$ in volume. The synthesis and secretion of angiogenic factors establish a vascular network from the surrounding stroma, the process called angiogenesis. Local invasion of some tumour cells to the host stroma occurs and the new blood vessels can provide the routes by which the cells leave the tumour and enter the blood circulation, which is termed intravasation. Tumour cells might also enter the circulation indirectly via the lymphatic system. The circulating cells arrest selectively in blood vessels of distant target organs, where the cells may migrate into the surrounding tissue, termed extravasation. In target organs, the cells are exposed to different types of homeostatic factors provided in the microenvironment, resulting in the formation and growth of secondary tumours, metastases. It is important to note that the process of tumour progression to metastasis is inherently inefficient, based on the evidence that only a few cells from primary tumours can complete the entire metastatic process [132]. Radioactive labelling of tumour cells has demonstrated that, within 24 hours after entry to blood circulation, less than 0.1% of tumour cells are still viable and less than 0.01% of the cells in the circulation survive to form metastases at the target sites [34]. The ability of these cells to successfully metastasize is dependent on both intrinsic properties of the tumour cells and normal host response in all steps of cancer progression [35].

Tumour Metastasis and the Hypothesis of "Seed" and "Soil"

Metastasis, a critical step of cancer progression, has been recognized as a non-random but highly organ-selective process. For example; in breast cancer, secondary tumours are usually found in the lung, liver, bone marrow and lymph nodes but rarely in other organs [128]. The first investigation of factors regulating certain patterns of cancer metastasis, known as the hypothesis of "seed" and "soil", dates back to 1889. Paget suggested that the metastasis occurred when tumour cells, referred to as the "seed", are compatible with a particular organ microenvironment, equated to the "soil". A review of this aspect shows that accumulating data mostly support Paget's hypothesis and provide a current definition of "seed" and "soil" theory [35, 36]. It has been suggested that primary tumours are inherently heterogeneous and contain subpopulations of cells with a variety of biological characteristics and only cancer cells with particular phenotypes including metastatic and invasive properties succeed in the formation of secondary tumours at the metastatic sites. The outcome of metastasis also appears to be dependent on multiple interactions between tumour cells and host homeostatic mechanisms, especially at the level of the microenvironment in target organs, where the initiation of secondary tumour growth preferentially occurs [20, 65]. In addition, three of the "fertile soil" concepts have recently been proposed to explain the preference of metastatic sites. Tumour cells randomly distribute throughout the body and will selectively proliferate at the sites producing appropriate growth factors, which support survival and proliferation of tumour cells; adhesion molecules, which specifically trap the circulating cells; and chemoattractants, which promote tumour cell homing to particular sites [57, 58, 71, 75].

Molecular Mechanisms of Cancer Metastatic Progression

Advances in molecular studies on mechanisms of cancer pathogenesis have led to the identification of a wide range of host factors that play important roles in the development of cancer. The majority of these molecules are the components of endocrine and immune systems that have become therapeutic targets for cancer [90, 96]. The most well-studied hormonal receptors, oestrogen receptor α and β isoforms (ERα and ERβ), and their involvement in the progression of cancer, particularly breast cancer, were discovered more than three decades ago. ERβ expression predominates in normal breast tissue, being detected in 22% of samples tested, whereas ERα is expressed in most tumours either alone or in combination with ERβ. The co-expression of the two isoforms is associated with a poor prognosis of breast cancer [113]. An increase in ERβ expression was also observed in chemically transformed human breast epithelial cells, implicating it in the process of carcinogenesis [45]. Numerous studies revealing the function of oestrogen and oestrogen receptors in breast cancer progression have led to the development of the first molecular-targeted breast cancer drug, tamoxifen, an antagonist of both oestrogen receptors [128]. This drug has been successful in treating approximately 60% of breast cancer with ERα-positive lesions; despite this many of these patients eventually develop recurrent cancers [112].

The family of growth factor receptor tyrosine kinases (RTKs) as well as their downstream signalling molecules has been implicated in cancer progression. As is the case for breast carcinoma, the approaches targeting several types of growth factor RTKs have been developed for treatment of the oestrogen receptor-negative cancers, which appear to be highly aggressive and are unresponsive to conventional anti-oestrogen therapy [3, 46, 78, 139]. Numerous studies have implicated HER2/ErbB2, a member of the epidermal growth factor receptor (EGFR) family, known as one of the most important oncoproteins, in breast tumourigenesis and metastasis [139]. Overexpression of the HER2/ErbB2 gene is found in human breast carcinomas, with a frequency of 25–30%, and also correlates with a more aggressive phenotype of breast cancer [108, 109, 135]. The first RTK-specific anti-oncogene drug, Herceptin, which inhibits the function of HER2/ErbB2, has been developed and is used currently for the treatment of HER2/ErbB2-positive breast cancer, with up to a 15% response rate [25]. The role of several other types of RTKs in breast cancer development has also been investigated. For example, EGFR/ErbB1 is also expressed in 14–91% of breast cancer. Its expression is a modest prognostic indicator and inversely correlates with oestrogen receptor status [51, 78]. The vascular endothelial growth factor receptors (VEGFRs), expressed on endothelial cells, appear to be key regulators of the formation of new vascular networks in tumours, termed angiogenesis, whereas the insulin-like growth factor (IGF) receptors have generated much interest due to their ability to inhibit programmed cell death, which is thought to function aberrantly during tumourigenesis, in addition to their established roles in oncogenic transformation and metastasis [46, 139]. Indeed, the roles of these growth factor RTKs are not limited to breast carcinoma, having been implicated in many other types of cancer including hepatocellular, ovarian, colorectal and prostate cancers. This has made these RTKs potential targets for cancer therapy [44].

A variety of molecules including mediators generated during the immune response to tumours are also known as important factors for the progression of cancer, especially inflammation-associated cancer. Proinflammatory cytokines such as interleukin-6 (IL-6) and tumour necrosis factor (TNF) have significant roles in inflammation-associated cancer [62]. Several lines of evidence indicate that IL-6 promotes tumour growth both *in vitro* and *in vivo* [17, 103], whereas TNF is known to have both anti- and pro-cancer actions [12]. TNF can induce

DNA damage, inhibit DNA repair and act as a growth factor for tumour cells [48]. Nonetheless, high-dose administration of TNF can destroy vasculature and therefore results in tumour necrosis [12]. The chemokines have recently generated much attention. To date, they have been implicated in transformation, growth, angiogenesis, invasion and metastasis of a number of types of cancer [121]. Several lines of evidence, both *in vitro* and *in vivo*, support the concept that certain chemokines act as tissue-specific attractant molecules for tumour cells, promoting the metastatic process of breast cancer [71, 73]. Due to prominent roles of the immune mediators in the progression of malignancy, further intensive investigations on this subject will provide a better understanding of the molecular pathogenesis of cancer.

Chemokines and Chemokine Receptors in Cancer Progression

Introduction

The chemokines, a superfamily of low molecular weight *chemo*tactic cyto*kines,* are well established as key regulators of leukocyte trafficking and other biological activities including development, angiogenesis and haematopoiesis. Chemokine action on leukocytes is associated with many cellular responses essential for cell migration including cytoskeleton rearrangement, cell polarization and integrin-dependent adhesion [11, 68], which are achieved through activation of G proteins and subsequent downstream effector kinases (Fig. 1). Nonetheless, it has become evident that they also participate in the activities of various types of other cells and contribute not only to homeostasis but also to many pathological conditions including cancer [11, 39, 121]. The expression of components of the chemokine family has been reported in a variety of human tumours and they have been identified as important mediators in the process of tumour progression to malignancy [7, 49, 121]. In the tumour microenvironment, specific chemokines have been shown to be responsible for the recruitment of leukocytes into the tumour sites. However, they may also play a role in the functionality of tumour cells and other surrounding cells in the microenvironment, which together regulate the process of cancer development [49]. Indeed, a number of pieces of evidence demonstrate the contribution of chemokines to multiple steps of tumour progression to malignancy, including tumourigenesis, growth/survival, angiogenesis, invasion and metastasis [7, 49, 121, 129]. Figure 2 summarizes the potential involvement of the chemokines in the progressive steps of cancer development.

Chemokines and the Tumour Immune Response

The microenvironment of the tumour is composed of tumour cells as well as various types of stromal cells such as fibroblasts and endothelial cells.

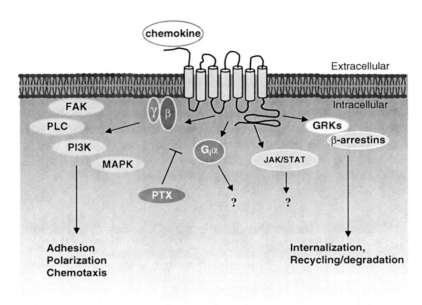

Fig. 1 Summary of major signal transduction pathways downstream of chemokine receptors. This simplified figure depicts signalling molecules activated following chemokine receptor activation. The binding of chemokines to their respective receptors results in the activation of three main downstream signalling pathways to various cellular responses. The classical G-protein pathway activates various downstream systems including PLC, PI3K, FAK and MAPK, leading to cell adhesion, polarization and chemotaxis. This pathway can be inhibited by inactivating Giα using PTX (*oval*). The activation of the JAK/STAT pathway being initiated following the tyrosine phosphorylation of activated chemokine receptors has been documented [68]. The signalling pathways initiated by phosphorylation at serine/threonine residues on the COOH-terminus region involve the activities of GRKs and β-arrestins. This pathway is responsible for internalization and recycling/degradation of the activated receptors. *Arrows* indicate "activated downstream". *Question marks* indicate unclear downstream signalling pathways. *FAK* focal adhesion kinase, *PLC* phospholipase C , *PI3K* phosphatidylinositol 3-kinase, *MAPK* mitogen-activated protein kinase, *PTX* pertussis toxin, *JAK/STAT* Janus kinase/Signal transducer and activator of transcription, *GRKs* G-protein-coupled receptor kinases. Modified from Mellado, M., Rodriguez-Frade, J. M., et al. (2001). Chemokine signaling and functional responses: the role of receptor dimerization and TK pathway activation. *Annu Rev Immunol* **19**: 397–421 and Thelen, M. (2001). Dancing to the tune of chemokines. *Nat Immunol* **2**(2): 129–34

Moreover, it is apparent that several types of inflammatory cells including neutrophils, macrophages and lymphocytes are recruited to the sites of tumour formation and these cells are suggested to play both positive and negative roles in the development of cancer [17, 18, 26, 49, 56, 79]. Accumulating data indicate that the infiltration of the inflammatory cells is regulated by a variety of biologically active molecules in the tumour microenvironment and the chemokines, in particular, play an important role in this process (reviewed in [49]). Thus, for example, ovarian cancer cells secrete some chemokines including

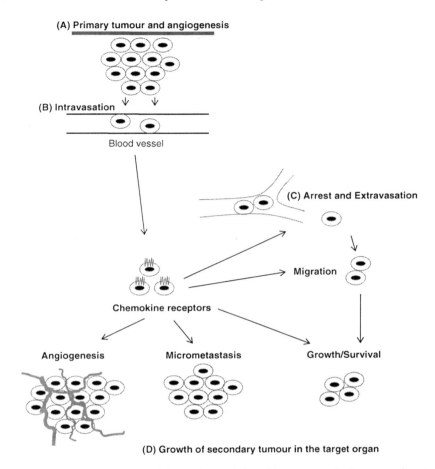

Fig. 2 The potential involvement of chemokines and chemokine receptors in the progressive steps of tumour progression to malignancy. The stepwise processes of cancer progression include (A) the initial transformation and growth at primary sites, the formation of a vascular network from surrounding tissue, a process called angiogenesis; (B) entry of tumour cells into the blood circulation, known as intravasation; (C) survival in the circulation, arrest in the target organs, penetration into surrounding tissue, termed extravasation; and (D) cell proliferation and secondary tumour growth at the sites of metastasis. Chemokines and chemokine receptors potentially play important roles in several steps of tumour progression, particularly the process of metastasis, including intravasation, arrest, extravasation, migration, growth/survival and micrometastasis and angiogenesis of the secondary tumour. Modified from Kakinuma, T. and Hwang S. T. (2006). Chemokines, chemokine receptors, and cancer metastasis. *J Leukoc Biol* **79**(4): 639–51

CCL2 [79]. CCL2 is found in tumour epithelial areas and there is a correlation between the number of cells expressing CCL2 and the total number of CD8$^+$ T lymphocytes and macrophages [79]. In oesophageal carcinoma, the expression of CCL2 is positively correlated with the level of macrophage infiltration, which also correlates with tumour angiogenesis [84]. CCL2 also induces the production of monocyte matrix metalloproteinases (MMPs), the matrix-degrading enzymes that are required for the extravasation of leukocytes through basement membrane into the tissue [94]. Similar to CCL2, the chemokine CCL5 is localized to areas containing tumour-infiltrating leukocytes and is responsible for the selective infiltration of T lymphocytes in human colorectal carcinoma [76]. Consequently, as demonstrated in numerous studies, different types of leukocytes recruited to tumour sites such as Th2 lymphocytes, immature dendritic cells, T regulatory cells and macrophages act in different manners to suppress or promote tumourigenesis [49].

Chemokines in Tumor Development, Growth and Angiogenesis

Evidence supports significant roles for chemokines, localized in the tumour microenvironment, in the processes of tumour formation and growth, and expression of a number of chemokine receptors has been associated with the process of tumourigenesis. CXCR2, the receptor for multiple inflammatory chemokines such as CXCL1 and CXCL8, demonstrates a high degree of homology to the GPCR encoded by Kaposi's sarcoma-associated herpes-virus-8, called KSHV-GPCR. A point mutation of CXCR2 results in the constitutive signalling of the receptors and cellular transformation in a manner similar to that by KSHV-GPCR [9, 19]. Overexpression of the ligands for CXCR2, CXCL2 and CXCL3 in melanocytes also increases their tumourigenicity *in vitro* and in nude mice [85]. A proliferative effect of chemokines on tumour cells has also been demonstrated. Two ligands for CXCR2, CXCL1 and CXCL8 have been identified as autocrine growth factors of melanoma cells, which constitutively express CXCR2. Blocking CXCL1 or CXCR2 function with specific antibodies inhibits melanoma cell growth [72, 83, 101]. In addition, some chemokines may support tumour growth by providing anti-apoptotic signals as shown by the evidence that CXCL12 and CXCL9 enhance the survival of tumour cells, expressing their cognate receptors CXCR4 and CXCR3, respectively, in serum-free conditions [50, 136].

Chemokines also affect the growth of tumours by regulating the formation of vascular networks from surrounding tissues. Particular types of CXC chemokines, containing an ELR (Glu-Leu-Arg) motif at the NH_2-terminus, appear to promote blood vessel growth in tumours. The ELR-positive chemokine CXCL8 elicits an angiogenic effect on prostate tumours. CXCL8 is found to be elevated in the serum of prostate cancer patients when compared with healthy subjects or patients with benign tumours and also in tissue samples of prostate cancer but not in normal or benign prostatic hyperplasia [33, 127]. The administration of a neutralizing antibody to CXCL8 inhibits tumour growth and tumour-related angiogenesis [70] in a SCID mouse model of human prostate cancer using prostate cancer cells, which constitutively produce CXCL8. Other ELR-positive CXC chemokines such as CXCL1, CXCL2 and CXCL3 also show angiogenic properties as demonstrated by experiments in which the overexpression of these chemokines in non-tumorigenic mouse melanocytes caused the formation of highly vascular tumours in mice [63, 85]. In contrast, ELR-negative CXC chemokines such as CXCL4, CXCL9 and CXCL10 show angiostatic activity, that is, they have the ability to inhibit angiogenesis [4, 6, 116]. In SCID mice, the intratumoural injection of CXCL10 attenuates the growth and neovascularization of non-small cell lung cancer, whereas blocking the function of CXCL10 by the administration of a specific neutralizing antibody enhances tumour growth and angiogenesis [5]. However, the ELR-negative CXC chemokine CXCL12 appears to exhibit angiogenic ability both *in vitro* and *in vivo* [42, 100]. Overall, it is believed that a balance between the activities of angiogenic and angiostatic factors, including certain CXC chemokines, is required for the formation of the neovascular network in tumours [6, 116].

Chemokines in Tumor Invasion and Metastasis

In recent years, the chemokines and their receptors have attracted much attention due to their significant roles in the late stages of cancer, metastasis and invasion. The function of these molecules in cancer spread has been inferred from the physiological activities of leukocytes especially that of chemotaxis, which is well known to be regulated by chemokines. In a seminal study by Muller et al. [73] it was suggested that metastasizing tumour cells migrate towards chemokine-producing secondary organs similar to the mechanisms for directional migration of leukocytes to sites of inflammation. Numerous further studies have demonstrated the involvement of various chemokines and chemokine receptors in metastasis and invasion of cancer [49]. Thus, expression of CXCL8 as well as its corresponding receptors, CXCR1 and CXCR2, increases the invasiveness of human melanoma cells and correlates with the metastatic potential of the cells in mice [107, 126]. Furthermore, overexpression of CXCL8 also results in an increase in invasion and metastasis, both *in vitro* and *in vivo* in a mouse model of prostate cancer [47]. CCR7, the receptor for CCL19 and CCL21, has also been implicated in melanoma metastasis. The functional expression of CCR7 enhances the metastasis of B16 murine melanoma cells, and this is inhibited by a neutralizing antibody to CCL21 [133]. A number of chemokines promote the invasive and metastatic potential of breast cancer cells. A wide range of ligands including CCL3, CCL4, CCL2, CCL5, CXCL10, CXCL7, CXCL1 and CXCL2 have been shown to induce the migration of human breast cancer cells [134]. The expression of CXCL8 has also been correlated with the metastatic potential of breast cancer cell lines [29].

The first experimental evidence revealing a molecular mechanism for chemokine-mediated organ-specific metastasis of breast cancer was reported by Muller and colleagues [73]. Amongst 17 different chemokine receptors, CXCR4 and CCR7 were predominantly expressed in human breast cancer cell lines, malignant breast tumours and metastases, compared with normal mammary epithelial cells. The functionality of CXCR4 and CCR7 was demonstrated by *in vitro* experiments showing that the stimulation of human breast cancer cells with CXCL12 and CCL21 mediates actin polymerization, chemotaxis and invasion. A panel of normal human organs was screened for the respective ligands: CXCL12 for CXCR4 and CCL21 for CCR7. It was found that CXCL12 was preferentially expressed at high levels in all target organs for breast cancer metastasis: the lung, liver, bone marrow, and lymph nodes and at low levels in all other organs. On the other hand, CCL21 was expressed selectively in lymph nodes. Protein extracts of the target organs exerted chemotactic activity on breast cancer cells. In a metastatic model of human breast cancer, involving injection of MDA-MB-231 cells, either orthotopically into the mammary fat pad or intravenously into immunodeficient SCID mice, blocking the interaction of CXCL12 and CXCR4 by the administration of a neutralizing antibody to CXCR4 attenuated metastasis to the regional lymph node and lung. This study indicates a significant involvement of CXCR4/CXCL12 and potentially CCR7/CCL21 in the development of breast cancer metastasis and invasion. Several more recent studies using different methods to block the activity of CXCR4 also support such a role. Downregulation of CXCR4 receptors by inducible small-interfering RNA (siRNA) inhibits the metastasis of breast cancer cells both *in vitro* and *in vivo* [24, 55], and blocking CXCR4 activity using a specific antagonist delays the growth of breast cancer cells in the lung [110]. The impact of CXCR4/CXCL12 on metastasis has also been reported by many studies in other types of metastatic cancers, including prostate, melanoma, pancreatic, and ovarian cancers [13, 14], and the CXCR4/CXCL12 axis is currently considered as one of the major determinants of cancer metastatic progression.

A number of recent reports have extensively investigated the biological functions of CXCR4/CXCL12 that are associated with the metastatic potential of cancer cells and several mechanisms underlying these processes have been suggested [49]. First, the activation of CXCR4 may trigger the arrest of circulating cancer cells on endothelial cells by promoting the interaction between adhesion molecules on both cell types. In B16 murine melanoma cells, the activation of CXCR4 rapidly increases the affinity of $\beta 1$ integrin on the cells for vascular cell adhesion molecule 1 (VCAM-1). Under shear stress conditions, overexpression of CXCR4 in B16 cells resulted in greater than tenfold increase in adhesion to lung endothelial cells expressing VCAM-1 in response to TNF-α [21]. Second, a cancer cell exploits CXCR4/CXCL12 to drive proliferation and survival. As demonstrated in many types of cancers, for example melanoma, glioma, and ovarian tumours, the stimulation by CXCL12 leads to an increase in proliferation and survival of CXCR4-expressing cancer cells [23, 74, 104, 136]. CXCR4/CXCL12 signal transduction leading to cell survival is likely to be mediated by the activation of PI3Ks and their downstream PKB/Akt [136]. Thirdly, the latest studies have demonstrated that the malignant transformation and the function of CXCR4 and CCR7 chemokine receptors are interconnected and, most importantly, are interdependent in breast cancer cells [43] (Kochetkova and McColl, unpublished) [2]. These latest advances in the understanding of the pathobiology of chemokine receptors in metastatic breast cancer cells are discussed below.

Cross-Talk Between Chemokines and Growth Factors in Cancer Progression

Tumour progression is known to be influenced by a variety of homeostatic factors released locally and systematically; for example adhesion molecules, immune components, and growth factors [58, 82, 106]. In the tumour–stroma interface, a tumour cell can be simultaneously exposed to a variety of humoral factors produced by both tumour and host cells. In recent years, it has become well documented that the families of G-protein-coupled receptors (GPCRs) and RTKs – two major groups of receptor proteins on the cell surface – play important roles in mediating the signals from extracellular stimuli such as hormones, growth factors and cytokines and the functions of both types of receptors are involved in a variety of physiological and pathological conditions [53, 114]. More importantly, recent studies have indicated that the signal transduction cascades mediated by the two receptor types share some downstream signalling pathways and may modulate each other to transduce the signals, a process termed cross-talk [64, 131]. Cross-talk between these receptors adds a significant complexity to their downstream signal transduction networks which translate multiple signals from extracellular stimulus into cellular activity and this may affect the physiological and pathological conditions mediated by the two types of receptors.

As mentioned above, several growth factor systems play crucial roles in cancer development, for example the EGF, VEGF and IGF families. These molecules have been identified as therapeutic targets for cancer therapy [53]. One of the well-established growth factor systems, the IGF family, has been documented to contribute to the processes of transformation, proliferation, survival and, lesser defined, invasion and metastasis, therefore controlling the accomplishment of malignant potential of tumour [37, 41, 99, 117]. Numerous molecular studies indicate that the activation of IGF tyrosine kinase receptor and chemokine CXCR4 receptor by their respective ligands, IGFs and CXCL12, respectively, triggers signal transduction pathways to cell migration which is a cellular activity mandatory for metastasis and invasion of cancer cells [37, 68]. Consequently, this significant contribution to the development of the invasion and metastasis of cancer, together with a documented cross-talk between signal transduction downstream of other GPCRs and that of RTKs reported in many cellular systems, prompted the investigation of potential cross-talk between IGF receptor and CXCR4.

IGF System in Breast Cancer Progression

The IGF system is extremely complex, comprising a number of ligands, binding proteins and receptors that can form homo- and heterodimers (Fig. 3A). With the exception of IGF-2, the receptors are multimeric, comprising 2α and 2β subunits (Fig. 3B). IGF-1R is an RTK with the β subunits containing the kinase domain. Ligand binding leads to activation of the kinase domain and subsequent activation of a number of downstream effector molecules (Fig. 4). IGFs contribute to the normal growth, development and survival in many tissue types. IGF-I, as an effector molecule of growth hormone action (GH), appears to be an endocrine factor promoting growth and development after birth and also plays a role as a local mediator involved in mammary gland development [41, 97, 99, 130]. However, accumulating evidence also suggests an association of the expression of IGF components with breast tumourigenesis. Several studies have shown significant overexpression of IGF-1R in cancer cells compared with normal and benign breast tissues [27, 86, 87]. A number of reports documented a role for IGFs and IGF-1R in breast cancer transformation, growth and survival [16, 17, 118, 119]. In addition, inhibition of IGF-1R expression by anti-sense-IGF-1R RNA, or its function by anti-IGF-1R antibody or dominant-negative mutants, resulted in slower growth and reduced transforming potential in various cell types including breast cancer cells [15, 41]. The tumourigenicity of IGF-1R is suggested to be related to hyperactivation of IGF-1R signal transduction, which can be caused by an overexpression of ligands, receptors, signalling molecules such as IRS and constitutive activation of the downstream signalling, PI3K/Akt pathways [67].

In the last 10 years the involvement of the IGF system in metastasis and invasion of various types of cancers including breast cancer has become increasingly evident [41, 60, 117]. In vitro studies have demonstrated that IGF-I elicits a chemotactic response from both non-metastatic MCF-7 and metastatic MDA-MB-231 human breast cancer cells and a neutralizing anti-IGF-1R inhibits IGF-I-induced chemotaxis in those cells [31, 2, 38, 52]. The inhibition of IGF-1R function by dominant-negative IGF-1R mutants suppresses adhesion, invasion and metastasis of breast cancer cells both *in vitro* and in a mouse model [32, 98]. Several recent studies have also suggested that IGF system components may play an important role in promoting some of the cellular phenotypes associated with invasive and metastatic potential of breast cancer cells such as angiogenic ability, cell–cell adhesion and cell migration [8, 41, 54, 125]. However, while the mechanisms of IGF-I- and IGF-1R-mediated

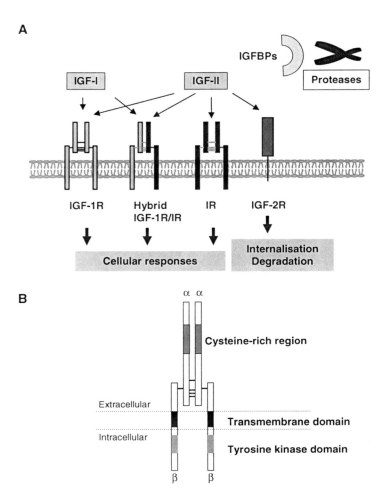

Fig. 3 Schematic representation of the IGF system (A) and structure of the IGF-1R (B). (A), The IGF system comprises a complex network of ligands (IGF-I and IGF-II), their cognate receptors (IGF-1R, IR, IGF-1R:IR hybrid, and IGF-2R) and six high-affinity IGFBPs and IGFBP proteases. IGFs are found circulating mainly in a complex containing IGFs and IGFBPs. Release of IGFs from the complex occurs upon IGFBP proteolysis or extracellular matrix (ECM) binding. This allows IGFs to bind to multiple cognate receptors with different affinities, mediating various biological responses [30]. (B), IGF-1R is a member of the receptor tyrosine kinase family, composed of two extracellular α subunits and two-membrane spanning β subunits. These subunits form a β−α−α−β arrangement and are held together by the α−α dimer and α−β disulfide bonds at the locations indicated [1]. *Black lines* indicate disulphide bridges. The major ligand-binding determinants are located within the α subunits. The intrinsic kinase domain, containing multiple sites of tyrosine phosphorylation, is located in the cytoplasmic portions of the β subunits. (A) is modified from Adams, T. E., Epa, V. C., et al. (2000). Structure and function of the type 1 insulin-like growth factor receptor. *Cell Mol Life Sci* **57**(7): 1050–93; Sachdev, D. and Yee, D. (2001). The IGF system and breast cancer. *Endocr Relat Cancer* **8**(3): 197–209; and Denley, A., Cosgrove, L. J., et al. (2005). Molecular interactions of the IGF system. *Cytokine Growth Factor Rev* **16**(4–5): 421–39, and (B) is modified from Adams, T. E., Epa, V. C., et al. (2000). Structure and function of the type 1 insulin-like growth factor receptor. *Cell Mol Life Sci* **57**(7): 1050–93

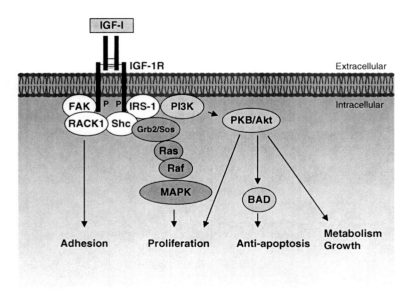

Fig. 4 Summary of the major signal transduction pathways downstream of IGF-1R This schematic depicts some of the established signalling molecules activated following the activation of IGF-1R [37, 99]. The binding of IGF-I to IGF-1R results in induction of intrinsic tyrosine kinase activity of the receptor. The phosphorylation of multiple tyrosine residues in the cytoplasmic portion of the receptor creates binding sites for several substrates including IRS-1, Shc, FAK and RACK1, which link IGF-1R to downstream signal transduction systems including PI3K and MAPK pathways, leading to various cellular activities. P indicates multiple phosphorylation on the cytoplasmic tail of IGF-1R. *IRS-1* insulin receptor substrate-1, *Shc* src-homology 2/2 α-collagen-related, *FAK* focal adhesion kinase, *RACK1* receptor for the activated C kinase 1, *Grb2* growth factor receptor-bound protein 2, *Sos* son of sevenless, *Raf* Ras activated factor, *MAPK* mitogen-activated protein kinases, PI3K phosphatidylinositol 3-kinase, *PKB/Akt* protein kinase B, and BAD bcl-associated death promoter

transformation and survival of tumour cells are relatively well studied, their function in the later stages of cancer disease, invasion and metastasis is not well understood.

Evidence for Cross-Talk Between CXCR4 and IGF-1R Signal Transduction in Breast Cancer Metastasis

CXCL12/CXCR4 and IGF-I/IGF-1R are well known as mediators for cellular activities such as proliferation, migration and anti-apoptosis. These ligand–receptor pairs are expressed in most cell types and tissues and contribute to a variety of physiological and pathological conditions. IGF-I/IGF-1R expression is of importance in growth and development of the foetus. A homozygous deletion of either IGF-I or IGF-1R gene in mice leads to decreased birth weight and the majority of mice die shortly after birth because of hypodevelopment of organs, particularly in the respiratory system [59]. CXCL12/CXCR4 plays a fundamental role in foetal development and naïve leukocyte trafficking. Mice in which CXCL12 or CXCR4 has been knocked out die in utero and are defective in many physiological systems including vascular development, haematopoiesis and cardiogenesis [77, 119, 138]. Certainly, these ligand–receptor systems share similarities in their physiological functions and this in itself suggests a potential contribution of the cross-talk between their signalling to these physiological outcomes.

As mentioned in the previous sections, both CXCR4 and IGF-1R have been independently shown to play crucial roles in tumour progression, particularly in the processes of invasion and metastasis of breast carcinoma. However, compared with leukocytes, the molecular mechanisms involved in activation of these receptors in epithelial cells are not well understood. Therefore, recent studies in our laboratory have begun to analyse the signal transduction downstream of chemokine GPCRs and IGF-1R RTK as well as their cross-talk in breast cancer cells [2, 43]. In order to relate our findings to the metastatic/invasive phenotype, we have compared the expression and function of the two receptors as well as the cross-talk between their signal transduction pathways in a panel of metastatic and non-metastatic breast epithelial cells. Initial studies focused on the highly metastatic MDA-MB-231 cells and the non-metastatic MCF-7 cells. While both cell lines expressed IGF-1R and CXCR4, the latter receptor was only active in the metastatic cell line (to be discussed in more detail later). In addition, it was shown that IGF-I transactivates CXCR4/G-protein signal transduction in MDA-MB-231 cells, but not in MCF-7 cells. Importantly, these studies show that the CXCR4/G-protein signalling apparatus in the highly metastatic MDA-MB-231 cells can also be utilized by IGF-I/IGF-1R [2].

The molecular basis for this novel cross-talk between CXCR4 and IGF-1R in a breast cancer epithelial cell has been examined. Based on the data obtained, a hypothetical model for interaction between these two receptors has been proposed (see Fig. 5). In the highly metastatic MDA-MB-231 cells, cross-talk between CXCR4 and IGF-1R occurs at the level of receptor/receptor interaction and appears to be unidirectional. While CXCL12 does not induce activation of IGF-1R, IGF-I is able to transactivate CXCR4/G-protein signal transduction in this cell type. It is apparent that this cross-talk is not mediated through a sequential or autocrine mechanism as supported by the fact that production and release of the ligand for CXCR4 and CXCL12 are not required for such transactivation. Rather, similar to the model for PDGFR/S1P$_1$ receptor interaction previously reported [91], co-immunoprecipitation studies indicate that the cross-talk between signal transduction of CXCR4 and IGF-1R depends on the physical formation of a complex containing IGF-1R, CXCR4 and G-proteins, $G_i\alpha_2$ and $G\beta$ (see Fig. 5A (1) and (2)). This receptor complex appears to be constitutively formed and probably provides a sufficiently close proximity of these proteins to allow IGF-I/IGF-1R to transactivate CXCR4 through release of $G_i\alpha$ and $G\beta$. These activation pathways apparently work

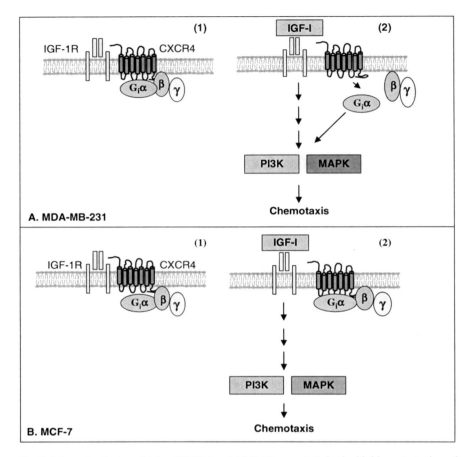

Fig. 5 A hypothetical model for CXCR4 and IGF-1R cross-talk in the highly metastatic and non-metastatic MCF-7 cells. The figure depicts signal transduction induced by IGF-I stimulation in MDA-MB-231 (**A**) and MCF-7 (**B**) cells in the resting state (1) and activation state (2). The constitutive formation of a signalling complex containing IGF-1R, CXCR4/G-proteins, $G_i\alpha$ and $G\beta\gamma$ is found in both MDA-MB-231 and MCF-7 cells (**A** and **B** (1)). In MDA-MB-231 cells (**A**), IGF-I can transactivate CXCR4/G-protein signalling pathways that work coordinately with tyrosine kinase-dependent pathways of IGF-1R to promote a chemotactic response of the cells (**A** (2)). The two major signalling systems, PI3K and MAPK, may be activated in this cross-talk. In MCF-7 cells (**B**), in contrast, there is no transactivation of CXCR4/G-protein signal transduction by IGF-I due to non-functional CXCR4 expressed in this cell type. Chemotaxis of MCF-7 cells induced by IGF-I may be dependent solely on tyrosine kinase-dependent pathways of IGF-1R (**B** (2)). *MAPK* mitogen-activated protein kinases,s *PI3K* phosphatidylinositol 3-kinase

together with a classical tyrosine kinase-dependent pathway downstream of IGF-I/IGF-1R to drive a chemotactic response of the cells. In MCF-7 cells, the physical association of IGF-1R and CXCR4/G-proteins is also found at the resting state (see Fig. 5B (1) and (2)). Nonetheless, IGF-I is unable to transactivate CXCR4/G-protein activation pathways due to non-functional CXCR4 in this cell line [2]. The defect of CXCR4 signalling in MCF-7 cells is found at the level of G-protein activation. Thus, chemotaxis of MCF-7 cells by IGF-I is presumably mediated only through IGF-1R tyrosine kinase-dependent pathways. The model for CXCR4/IGF-1R interaction described here clearly shows how IGF-1R and CXCR4 coordinately activate signal transduction, leading to a migrational response of the highly metastatic MDA-MB-231 cells [2].

While the existence of the cross-talk between CXCR4 and IGF-1R in breast cancer cells and its potential contribution to an acquisition of metastatic and invasive phenotypes of breast cancer have been reported, further investigation of molecular mechanisms underlining the establishment of the cross-talk is required. One of the hypotheses for the formation of cross-talk between signal transduction mediated by different receptor types is based on the concept of lipid raft formation. In the past decade, several lines of evidence have increasingly supported that signal transduction initiated by receptors on the cell surface in response to extracellular stimuli is influenced by formation of membrane microdomains, enriched in cholesterol and glycosphingolipids, termed lipid rafts. Lipid rafts containing a set of membrane signalling proteins have been considered as a platform that mediates intracellular signal transduction [89, 105]. Currently, a number of GPCRs and RTKs have been shown to be associated with lipid rafts, which is obligatory for ligand–receptor binding and receptor signalling [88]. While the disruption of lipid raft structure by cholesterol depletion inhibits ligand binding to the receptors and impairs the ability of receptors to mediate signalling, replenishment of cell membrane with cholesterol effectively restores the receptor ability to transduce signals [81, 93]. It is hypothesized that rafts contain a distinctive protein and lipid composition that is important to accomplish specific signalling functions. It is also possible that establishment of lipid rafts may be responsible for transactivation among different types of receptors especially between GPCRs and RTKs. This is the case for transactivation of PDGFR and EGFR by the GPCR ligand, S1P. It appears that the transactivation is abolished by depletion of cholesterol, suggesting requirement of the cholesterol-rich microdomains for this cross-activation [122]. Both CXCR4 and IGF-1R are raft-associated proteins and their ability to mediate signalling is also supported by lipid raft formation [81, 93]. As discussed above, the cross-talk between CXCR4 and IGF-1R signalling observed in MDA-MB-231 cells is based on the formation of a signalling complex containing IGF-1R, CXCR4 and CXCR4-associated proteins. The complex allows IGF-I to transduce signal transduction pathways of both IGF-1R and CXCR4 to cell migration. While mechanisms by which these proteins are recruited to form the complex are largely unclear, it is likely that lipid rafts support the establishment of this GPCR/RTK signalling complex.

Functional Relationship between Chemokine Receptors and the Metastatic Phenotype of Breast Cancer Cells

Expression of Chemokine Receptors and Cancer Metastasis

The expression of chemokine receptors CXCR4 and CCR7 in particular, on tumour cells has recently received a great deal of attention due to the discovery of their direct involvement in promoting cancer metastasis and their potential as metastatic markers. Expression of these chemokine receptors has been reported on a number of cancer cell lines, tissues and primary tumours and interaction with their specific ligands has been demonstrated to stimulate migration of cancer cells *in vitro* and *in vivo*. Of particular importance are retrospective studies in clinical samples, which use the expression of these chemokine receptors to correlate the outcome for cancer patients. Thus, the presence of CCR7 in non-small cell lung cancer (NSCLC) cells has been directly associated with the development of lymph node metastasis [120]. More specifically, CCR7 mRNA was expressed at higher levels in cancer tissue and not in the neighbouring normal lung tissues. Furthermore, the expression of CCR7 mRNA correlated with the stage of lymphatic invasion suggesting that CCR7 may participate in the emigration of cancer cells from peripheral tissue to lymph nodes via lymphatics. As a consequence, it was proposed that CCR7 expression could be used as a potential diagnostic tool for predicting lymph node metastasis before surgery and may improve disease-treatment planning of NSCLC. Since CXCR4 is the most common chemokine receptor expressed by tumour cells, being implicated in over 25 different epithelial, mesenchymal and haemopoietic human cancers [13, 14], its expression has been extensively studied in a large variety of tumour cells and tissues. Notably, not all cancer cells studied are CXCR4-positive. Some of the cell lines derived from ovarian cancer, acute myelogenous leukaemia (AML), anaplastic thyroid cancer and glioma are CXCR4-negative as are primary cells from acute myeloid AML, erythroid AML and undifferentiated AML [13, 14]. Moreover, within primary tumours such as ovary and NSCLC, only a subpopulation of cells expresses CXCR4. More importantly, CXCR4 expression has been linked to promoting the production of other factors that are involved in the processes of malignancy. For example, CXCL12 stimulation of ovarian cancer cell lines and primary cells isolated from ascitic disease caused production of the pro-inflammatory cytokine TNF-α [104], which has been implicated in tumour/stromal communication in this disease.

The majority of these studies has focused on positively correlating receptor expression with the metastatic disease state. However, conflicting evidence shows that the expression of CXCR4 on cancer cells is not simply confined to tumour cells exhibiting metastatic abilities. One study shows that CXCR4 expression was initiated at a very early point in the transition from normal to a transformed phenotype in breast epithelium, being highly expressed in ductal carcinoma *in situ* (DCIS), a precursor of invasive ductal carcinomas [102]. Moreover, high levels of CXCR4 were detected in 94% of studied cases of atypical ductal hyperplasia, potentially the first clonal pre-neoplastic expansion of ductal epithelial cells, representing an early stage in tumourigenic transformation [102]. Therefore, these observations raise the possibility that expression of important chemokine receptors implicated in metastasis, such as CXCR4 and CCR7, is not restricted to the more malignant forms of breast cancer.

In view of these contrasting data, the precise relationship of chemokine receptor expression in cancer cells and their potential role in metastatic tumour progression is still not clear and requires considerable clarification. To establish if the level of chemokine receptor expression relates to the disease stage of breast cancer, the analysis of CXCR4 and CCR7 expression in breast cancer cells was performed *in vitro* in a panel of cell lines ranging from non-transformed immortalized breast epithelial cells to highly aggressive breast cancer cell lines [43] (Kochetkova and McColl, unpublished). The examination of CXCR4 and CCR7 expression revealed significant levels of expression throughout the panel of breast epithelial cancer cell lines. CXCR4 and CCR7 expression were not restricted to the metastatic cell types with MCF10A cells, a non-transformed immortalized breast cancer cell line, exhibiting similar levels to that observed in highly invasive transformed breast cancer cell line, MDA-MB-231. These data challenge previous reports and strongly suggest that CXCR4 and CCR7 expression alone is not an indicator of aggressive breast cancer and therefore its application as a prognostic marker of metastasis requires extensive further clarification.

Functional Activation of Chemokine Receptors and Cancer Metastasis

The assessment of chemokine receptor functionality *in vitro* is routinely performed by measuring the ability of chemokine ligands to induce calcium mobilization, actin polymerization and chemotaxis, which are early physiological changes associated with chemokine receptor activation [28, 68]. These cellular responses were used to investigate the function of chemokine receptors in a large panel of breast cancer cells ranging from untransformed, immortalized breast epithelial to highly invasive, metastatic lines [43] (Kochetkova and McColl, unpublished). The biological significance of CXCR4 and CCR7 expression throughout this cell panel revealed a clear distinction in terms of responsiveness, with the specific chemokine ligands eliciting functional responses in the highly metastatic breast cancer cells but not in the non-metastatic cells. Radio-ligand binding assays revealed a similar number of receptors as well as ligand-binding affinities on metastatic and non-metastatic cells. Since these parameters were similar in all cell types, the observed differential receptor activation could not be accounted for and it was concluded that lack of functional receptor activity was probably attributed to a disruption in chemokine-mediated intracellular signalling.

The phenomenon of non-functional chemokine receptor expression is not common in the literature although there have been several examples described. In a recent study, Trentin et al. reported differential function of CXCR4 and other chemokine receptors in non-Hodgkin lymphomas [124]. Their findings revealed the expression of non-responsive CXCR4 in normal B cells (with respect to chemotaxis and calcium mobilization) and fully functional receptors in leukemic cells, similar to that observed for breast cancer cells. In a different study, an early signalling defect in the CXCR4-expressing hepatocellular carcinoma cell line, HepG2, was identified [69]. In those cells, CXCL12 was shown to bind to CXCR4 in Hep2G cells although the activation of downstream signalling events was not triggered. However, the transfection of exogenous CXCR4 into the Hep2G cell line was able to restore function upon CXCL12 treatment resulting in phosphorylation of p44/42, indicating the presence of intact signalling machinery in HepG2 cells transfected with CXCR4. A subpopulation of neuronal cells, cerebellar granule cells, has been reported to express non-functional CXCR4 while glial cells and cortical neurons were able to undergo chemotaxis and mobilize calcium in response to CXCL12 [10]. Finally, differences in CXCR4 functionality have been reported in normal and malignant human haematopoietic cells [66]. It was demonstrated that the activation of CXCR4 in human T-cell lines (Jurkat and ATL-2) rapidly induced phosphorylation of mitogen-activated protein kinases (MAPK) (p44 ERK-1 and p42 ERK-2). The CXCR4-mediated signalling in normal haematopoietic cells, human megakaryoblasts, which highly express CXCR4 as a model, also led to the phosphorylation of MAPK and serine/threonine kinase AKT after CXCL12 treatment. However, neither MAPK nor AKT was phosphorylated in normal human platelets after stimulation by CXCL12.

These findings strongly point to the existence of distinct mechanisms regulating the activation of CXCR4 and CCR7, which is likely to be cell type dependent. In the case of cancer progression, it is feasible to predict that cells that acquire functional chemokine receptors receive selective advantages to survive, migrate, invade and proliferate at secondary tumour sites. At this point in time, the physiological function of CXCR4 or CCR7 expression in non-metastatic breast cancer cells is not known, nor is it known for normal breast epithelial cells. However, the determination of their role would be valuable but to achieve this, further experiments will be required.

Molecular Mechanisms of the Functional On-Switch of the Chemokine Receptors in Metastatic Cancer Cells

There has been a great deal of interest in chemokine receptor signalling in cancer in terms of the specific pathways and effector molecules that regulate cell survival, proliferation, chemotaxis, migration and adhesion. It is clear that a large number of downstream effector molecules that are regulated by chemokines may account for the multiple effects of these receptors in the pathobiology of tumours. However, at this stage the role of various effectors of chemokine receptors in primary and metastatic tumours has not been well established. Moreover, investigations into chemokine signalling have predominantly been conducted in leukocytes with little evidence presently available on signalling cascades in cell types other than leukocytes. Major signalling pathways that are activated downstream of chemokine receptors are summarized in Fig. 1.

Although at the present time, relatively little is known regarding the signalling pathways activated by chemokines in cancer cells, preliminary data show that CXCR4 and CCR7 are capable of activating a number of different intracellular events such as chemotaxis, invasion and adhesion, all of which are properties that correlate with metastatic behaviour of tumour cells [40, 95].

As actin polymerization and chemotactic responses are not induced following the binding of CXCR4 and CCR7 ligands in non-metastatic breast cancer cells, it is possible that the signalling intermediates further upstream of these events are disrupted. Chemokine signalling pathways are mediated through GPCRs and generally use the Gi subclass of G proteins [137] that results in the activation of the Gαi subunit which mediates the inhibition of adenylyl cyclase-mediated cAMP production and the mobilization of intracellular calcium [80]. Treatment with CXCL12 or CCL19 inhibited forskolin-induced adenylyl cyclase-mediated cAMP in metastatic breast cancer cell lines; however, this was not the case for the non-metastatic cells. In addition chemokines induce Gαi-dependent intracellular calcium mobilization in metastatic breast cancer cells since it can be inhibited by pretreatment with pertussis toxin, an inhibitor of Gαi.

In cell types such as leucocytes, the $\beta\gamma$ subunit of the G-protein complex is responsible for the activation of numerous kinase cascades downstream of GPCRs [61]. In metastatic breast cancer cells a rapid and sustained activation of ERK1/2, IκBα, JNK, Akt, p38MAPK and GSK-3α/β was observed in response to CXCR4 and CCR7 ligands, while little to no activation was detected in any of the non-metastatic representative cell lines. Because several of these effector molecules play a significant role during the migration of leukocytes, these data imply that breast cancer cells use similar chemokine-mediated mechanisms to regulate processes such as migration, proliferation, survival and also metastasis. Moreover, the fact that G$\beta\gamma$-dependent signalling is not activated in the non-metastatic cell types suggests that the block in functional signalling occurs further upstream of these signalling intermediates. Overall, the analysis of the chemokine-mediated signalling events downstream of the G-protein α and $\beta\gamma$ subunits in breast cancer cells suggested that the blockade of CXCR4 and CCR7 function in non-metastatic cells occurs at the level of G protein activation.

Heterotrimeric G proteins act as molecular switches in signalling pathways by coupling the activation of heptahelical receptors at the cell surface to intracellular responses. This role depends on the ability of the Gα subunit to cycle between a resting conformation primed for interaction with an activated receptor and a signalling conformation capable of modulating the activity of downstream effector proteins. In the resting state, the Gα subunit binds GDP and $G\beta\gamma$. Receptors activate G proteins by catalysing GTP for GDP exchange on the $G\alpha$ subunit, leading to a conformational change in the $G\alpha$ and $G\beta\gamma$ subunits that allows their dissociation and activation of a variety of downstream effector proteins. The G protein returns to the resting conformation following GTP hydrolysis and subunit re-association.

Analysis of the chemokine receptor and G-protein coupling, examined in resting and chemokine-activated metastatic and non-metastatic breast cancer cells, demonstrated that CXCR4 and CCR7 formed complexes with the $G\alpha i$ subunit constitutively in both cell types. However, following chemokine stimulation, the dissociation of $G\alpha i$ from the receptor occurred only in the metastatic cells. In parallel, the $G\beta$ subunit associated with chemokine receptors in both non-invasive and metastatic breast cancer cells; however, the dissociation of $G\beta$ from the receptor upon ligand stimulation occurred only in the metastatic cells. Further investigations revealed that the formation of the heterotrimeric G-protein complex could only be detected in the invasive cell types that express functional chemokine receptors. The differences in $G\alpha_i$ and $G\beta$ binding observed throughout the panel of breast cancer cells lines were not due to the absence of $G\beta$ protein since all cells examined expressed $G\beta$ subunits. Therefore, this novel finding indicates that in non-invasive cells with non-functional CXCR4 or CCR7, $G\alpha_i$ and $G\beta\gamma$ do not form the functional heterotrimeric structure which is critical for GDP to GTP transfer and thus activation of signalling pathways downstream of G proteins [92].

These findings strongly suggest the existence of specific regulatory mechanisms that may be switched on or off during the metastatic progression of breast cancer which may have potentially important implications for the acquisition of an invasive, metastatic phenotype by the cells of breast and possibly other tumours. The hypothetical functional "on-switch" for chemokine receptors expressed in breast cancer cells is controlled at the level of the receptor and G-protein subunit interactions with CXCR4 and/or CCR7. The lack of the formation of the G-protein heterotrimeric complex in the non-invasive cells may be due to the expression of "incompatible" α and $\beta\gamma$ subunits in those cells. It is of note that the family of heterotrimeric G proteins consists of 27α, 5β and 14γ subunits, which leads to a very high number of possible $\alpha\beta\gamma$ subunit combinations of varying affinity for a multitude of GPCRs [136]. Another plausible explanation for the inability of $G\alpha$ and $G\beta\gamma$ subunits to form stable complexes in selective cell lines may be the expression of one or more inhibitory molecules. Of relevance, Soriano et al. recently found that SOCS3 upregulation by cytokines led to functional inactivation of CXCR4 via blockade of the $G\alpha_i$ pathway [111]. Specifically, SOCS3 overexpression stimulated by cytokines impaired the response to CXCL12 as determined by cell migration in *in vitro* and *in vivo* experiments. It was proposed that this effect is mediated by SOCS3 binding to the CXCR4, thereby blocking JAK/STAT and $G\alpha_i$ pathways.

Many aspects of G-protein-mediated signalling remain to be elucidated, and to gain a broader understanding of the functional roles of chemokine receptor signalling pathways in human breast and potentially other cancer cells, additional studies are necessary to delineate the regulation of G-proteins downstream of CXCR4 and CCR7. A detailed understanding of the physiological and pathophysiological role of G-protein-mediated signalling in normal and transformed cells will allow the full exploitation of this multifaceted signalling system as a target for pharmacological interventions.

Conclusion and Perspective

Cancer research has emphasized the importance not only of intrinsic properties of tumours but also of the host homeostatic systems activated during the process of cancer progression. Accumulating evidence has recently implicated the chemoattractant cytokines, named chemokines, which are major mediators in leukocyte trafficking and therefore regulate normal immune responses, in almost every step of cancer progression, particularly invasion and metastasis. Importantly, chemokines are believed to participate in the tumour microenvironment and potentially interact with growth factors to regulate the process of invasion and metastasis of cancer.

As thoroughly reviewed, molecular analyses have indicated that the activation of chemokine receptors by chemokines triggers the signal transduction networks leading to a migrational response which is mandatory for the accomplishment of invasive and metastatic ability of cancer cells. While different types of cross-talk between GPCR and RTK signal transduction are increasingly documented, it has been clearly demonstrated that the migrational signalling downstream of chemokine receptors can be transactivated by growth factors as is the case for the cross-talk between CXCR4/CXCL12 and IGF-1R/IGF-I in metastatic breast cancer cells. Despite the existence of cross-talk between the two types of receptors being documented, many important aspects require further investigation. Of importance, a variety of normal and diseased cells and tissues, including cancer cells other than those derived from breast cancer, should be examined for similar cross-talk. Different factors involved in establishing the CXCR4/IGF-1R signalling complex must be identified in order to elucidate the precise mechanism of the cross-talk. The role of this cross-talk in the development of breast cancer metastasis and invasion would also need to be studied in *in vivo* models once specific approaches to inhibit the cross-talk are available. Currently, cross-talk between different types of molecules exerting their biological effects on a tumour cell is being increasingly studied and this aspect is essential for an understanding in molecular pathogenesis of cancer that may lead to the development of effective cancer therapy.

Finally, the results of our studies demonstrating a disconnection between CXCR4 expression and function in breast cancer cells requires further evaluation. At first glance, they indicate that assessment of CXCR4 expression as a diagnostic of metastatic potential may not be appropriate, unless the approach incorporates evaluation of functional status. However, and perhaps of greater interest, is the possibility of uncovering the molecular mechanism behind inhibition of CXCR4 function in non-metastatic cells which may open the door to a new therapeutic approach to inhibit metastatic cells.

References

1. Adams, T. E., Epa, V. C., et al. (2000). Structure and function of the type 1 insulin-like growth factor receptor. *Cell Mol Life Sci* **57**(7): 1050–93.
2. Akekawatchai, C., Holland, J. D., et al. (2005). Transactivation of CXCR4 by the insulin-like growth factor-1 receptor (IGF-1R) in human MDA-MB-231 breast cancer epithelial cells. *J Biol Chem* **280**(48): 39701–8. Epub 2005 Sep 19.
3. Andrechek, E. R. and Muller, W. J. (2000). Tyrosine kinase signalling in breast cancer: tyrosine kinase-mediated signal transduction in transgenic mouse models of human breast cancer. *Breast Cancer Res* **2**(3): 211–6.
4. Angiolillo, A. L., Sgadari, C., et al. (1995). Human interferon-inducible protein 10 is a potent inhibitor of angiogenesis in vivo. *J Exp Med* **182**(1): 155–62.
5. Arenberg, D. A., Kunkel, S. L., et al. (1996). Interferon-gamma-inducible protein 10 (IP-10) is an angiostatic factor that inhibits human non-small cell lung cancer (NSCLC) tumorigenesis and spontaneous metastases. *J Exp Med* **184**(3): 981–92.
6. Arenberg, D. A., Polverini, P. J., et al. (1997). The role of CXC chemokines in the regulation of angiogenesis in non-small cell lung cancer. *J Leukoc Biol* **62**(5): 554–62.
7. Arya, M., Patel, H. R., et al. (2003). Chemokines: Key players in cancer. *Curr Med Res Opin* **19**(6): 557–64.
8. Bae, M. H., Lee, M. J., et al. (1998). Insulin-like growth factor II (IGF-II) secreted from HepG2 human hepatocellular carcinoma cells shows angiogenic activity. *Cancer Lett* **128**(1): 41–6.
9. Bais, Santomasso, C., B., et al. (1998). G-protein-coupled receptor of Kaposi's sarcoma-associated herpesvirus is a viral oncogene and angiogenesis activator. *Nature* **391**(6662): 86–9.
10. Bajetto, A., Bonavia, R., et al. (1999). Glial and neuronal cells express functional chemokine receptor CXCR4 and its natural ligand stromal cell-derived factor 1. *J Neurochem* **73**(6): 2348–57.
11. Balkwill, F. (1998). The molecular and cellular biology of the chemokines. *J Viral Hepat* **5**(1): 1–14.
12. Balkwill, F. (2002). Tumor necrosis factor or tumor promoting factor? *Cytokine Growth Factor Rev* **13**(2): 135–41.
13. Balkwill, F. (2004). Cancer and the chemokine network. *Nat Rev Cancer* **4**(7): 540–50.
14. Balkwill, F. (2004). The significance of cancer cell expression of the chemokine receptor CXCR4. *Semin Cancer Biol* **14**(3): 171–9.
15. Baserga (1995)
16. Baserga, R., Peruzzi, F. et al. (2003). The IGF-1 receptor in cancer biology. *Int J Cancer* **107**(6): 873–7.
17. Becker, C., Fantini, M. C., et al. (2004). TGF-beta suppresses tumor progression in colon cancer by inhibition of IL-6 trans-signaling. *Immunity* **21**(4): 491–501.
18. Brigati, C.,. Noonan, D. M., et al. (2002). Tumors and inflammatory infiltrates: friends or foes? *Clin Exp Metastasis* **19**(3): 247–58.
19. Burger, M., Burger, J. A., et al. (1999). Point mutation causing constitutive signaling of CXCR2 leads to transforming activity similar to Kaposi's sarcoma herpesvirus-G protein-coupled receptor. *J Immunol* **163**(4): 2017–22.

20. Cameron, M. D., Schmidt, E. E., et al. (2000). Temporal progression of metastasis in lung: cell survival, dormancy, and location dependence of metastatic inefficiency. *Cancer Res* **60**(9): 2541–6.
21. Cardones, A. R., Murakami, T., et al. (2003). CXCR4 enhances adhesion of B16 tumor cells to endothelial cells in vitro and in vivo via beta(1) integrin. *Cancer Res* **63**(20): 6751–7.
22. Chambers, A. F., Groom, A. C., et al. (2002). Dissemination and growth of cancer cells in metastatic sites. *Nat Rev Cancer* **2**(8): 563–72.
23. Chen, G. S., Yu, H. S., et al. (2006). CXC chemokine receptor CXCR4 expression enhances tumorigenesis and angiogenesis of basal cell carcinoma. *Br J Dermatol* **154**(5): 910–8.
24. Chen, Y., Stamatoyannopoulos, G., et al. (2003). Down-regulation of CXCR4 by inducible small interfering RNA inhibits breast cancer cell invasion in vitro. *Cancer Res* **63**(16): 4801–4.
25. Cobleigh, M. A., Vogel, C. L., et al. (1999). Multinational study of the efficacy and safety of humanized anti-HER2 monoclonal antibody in women who have HER2-overexpressing metastatic breast cancer that has progressed after chemotherapy for metastatic disease. *J Clin Oncol* **17**(9): 2639–48.
26. Coussens, L. M. and Werb Z. (2002). Inflammation and cancer. *Nature* **420**(6917): 860–7.
27. Cullen, K. J., Yee, D., et al. (1990). Insulin-like growth factor receptor expression and function in human breast cancer. *Cancer Res* **50**(1): 48–53.
28. Curnock, A. P., Logan, M. K., et al. (2002). Chemokine signalling: pivoting around multiple phosphoinositide 3-kinases. *Immunology* **105**(2): 125–36.
29. De Larco, J. E., Wuertz, B. R., et al. (2001). A potential role for interleukin-8 in the metastatic phenotype of breast carcinoma cells. *Am J Pathol* **158**(2): 639–46.
30. Denley, A., Cosgrove, L. J., et al. (2005). Molecular interactions of the IGF system. *Cytokine Growth Factor Rev* **16**(4–5): 421–39.
31. Doerr (1996)
32. Dunn, S. E., Ehrlich, M., et al. (1998). A dominant negative mutant of the insulin-like growth factor-I receptor inhibits the adhesion, invasion, and metastasis of breast cancer. *Cancer Res* **58**(15): 3353–61.
33. Ferrer, F. A., Miller, L. J., et al. (1998). Angiogenesis and prostate cancer: in vivo and in vitro expression of angiogenesis factors by prostate cancer cells. *Urology* **51**(1): 161–7.
34. Fidler, I. J. (1970). Metastasis: guantitative analysis of distribution and fate of tumor embolilabeled with 125 I-5-iodo-2'-deoxyuridine. *J Natl Cancer Inst* **45**(4): 773–82.
35. Fidler, I. J. (2002). The organ microenvironment and cancer metastasis. *Differentiation* **70** (9–10): 498–505.
36. Fidler, I. J. (2003). Timeline: The pathogenesis of cancer metastasis: the 'seed and soil' hypothesis revisited. *Nat Rev Cancer* **3**(6): 453–8.
37. Foulstone, E., Prince, S., et al. (2005). Insulin-like growth factor ligands, receptors, and binding proteins in cancer. *J Pathol* **205**(2): 145–53.
38. Furukawa, M., Raffeld, M., et al. (2005). Increased expression of insulin-like growth factor I and/or its receptor in gastrinomas is associated with low curability, increased growth, and development of metastases. *Clin Cancer Res* **11**(9): 3233–42.
39. Gale, L. M. and McColl, S. R. (1999). Chemokines: extracellular messengers for all occasions? *Bioessays* **21**(1): 17–28.
40. Ganju, R. K., Brubaker, S. A., et al. (1998). The alpha-chemokine, stromal cell-derived factor-1alpha, binds to the transmembrane G-protein-coupled CXCR-4 receptor and activates multiple signal transduction pathways. *J Biol Chem* **273**(36): 23169–75.
41. Gross, J. M. and Yee, D. (2003). The type-1 insulin-like growth factor receptor tyrosine kinase and breast cancer: biology and therapeutic relevance. *Cancer Metastasis Rev* **22**(4): 327–36.
42. Gupta, S. K., Lysko, P. G., et al. (1998). Chemokine receptors in human endothelial cells. Functional expression of CXCR4 and its transcriptional regulation by inflammatory cytokines. *J Biol Chem* **273**(7): 4282–7.

43. Holland, J. D., Kochetkova, M., et al. (2006). Differential functional activation of chemokine receptor CXCR4 is mediated by G proteins in breast cancer cells. *Cancer Res* **66**(8): 4117–24.
44. Hopfner, M., Schuppan, D. et al. (2008). Growth factor receptors and related signalling pathways as targets for novel treatment strategies of hepatocellular cancer. *World J Gastroenterol* **14**(1): 1–14.
45. Hu, Y. F., Lau, K. M., et al. (1998). Increased expression of estrogen receptor beta in chemically transformed human breast epithelial cells. *Int J Oncol* **12**(6): 1225–8.
46. Hynes, N. E. (2000). Tyrosine kinase signalling in breast cancer. *Breast Cancer Res* **2**(3): 154–7. Epub 2000 Apr 17.
47. Inoue, K., Slaton, J. W., et al. (2000). Interleukin 8 expression regulates tumorigenicity and metastases in androgen-independent prostate cancer. *Clin Cancer Res* **6**(5): 2104–19.
48. Jaiswal, M., LaRusso, N. F., et al. (2000). Inflammatory cytokines induce DNA damage and inhibit DNA repair in cholangiocarcinoma cells by a nitric oxide-dependent mechanism. *Cancer Res* **60**(1): 184–90.
49. Kakinuma, T. and Hwang S. T. (2006). Chemokines, chemokine receptors, and cancer metastasis. *J Leukoc Biol* **79**(4): 639–51.
50. Kawada, K., Sonoshita, M., et al. (2004). Pivotal role of CXCR3 in melanoma cell metastasis to lymph nodes. *Cancer Res* **64**(11): 4010–7.
51. Klijn, J. G., Berns, P. M., et al. (1992). The clinical significance of epidermal growth factor receptor (EGF-R) in human breast cancer: a review on 5232 patients. *Endocr Rev* **13**(1): 3–17.
52. Kornprat, P., Rehak, P., et al. (2006). Expression of IGF-I, IGF-II, and IGF-IR in gallbladder carcinoma. A systematic analysis including primary and corresponding metastatic tumours. *J Clin Pathol* **59**(2): 202–6.
53. Krause, D. S. and Van Etten R. A. (2005). Tyrosine kinases as targets for cancer therapy. *N Engl J Med* **353**(2): 172–87.
54. Lee, O. H., Bae, S. K., et al. (2000). Identification of angiogenic properties of insulin-like growth factor II in in vitro angiogenesis models. *Br J Cancer* **82**(2): 385–91.
55. Liang, Z., Yoon, Y.,et al. (2005). Silencing of CXCR4 blocks breast cancer metastasis. *Cancer Res* **65**(3): 967–71.
56. Lin, E. Y. and Pollard J. W. (2004). Role of infiltrated leucocytes in tumour growth and spread. *Br J Cancer* **90**(11): 2053–8.
57. Liotta, L. A. (2001). An attractive force in metastasis. *Nature* **410**(6824): 24–5.
58. Liotta, L. A. and. Kohn E. C (2001). The microenvironment of the tumour-host interface. *Nature* **411**(6835): 375–9.
59. Liu, J. P., Baker, J., et al. (1993). Mice carrying null mutations of the genes encoding insulin-like growth factor I (Igf-1) and type 1 IGF receptor (Igf1r). *Cell* **75**(1): 59–72.
60. Long, L., Rubin, R., et al. (1995). Loss of the metastatic phenotype in murine carcinoma cells expressing an antisense RNA to the insulin-like growth factor receptor. *Cancer Res* **55**(5): 1006–9.
61. Lopez-Ilasaca, M. (1998). Signaling from G-protein-coupled receptors to mitogen-activated protein (MAP)-kinase cascades. *Biochem Pharmacol* **56**(3): 269–77.
62. Lu, H., Ouyang, W., et al. (2006). Inflammation, a key event in cancer development. *Mol Cancer Res* **4**(4): 221–33.
63. Luan, J., Shattuck-Brandt, R., et al. (1997). Mechanism and biological significance of constitutive expression of MGSA/GRO chemokines in malignant melanoma tumor progression. *J Leukoc Biol* **62**(5): 588–97.
64. Luttrell, L. M., Daaka, Y., et al. (1999). Regulation of tyrosine kinase cascades by G-protein-coupled receptors. *Curr Opin Cell Biol* **11**(2): 177–83.
65. Luzzi, K. J., MacDonald, I. C., et al. (1998). Multistep nature of metastatic inefficiency: dormancy of solitary cells after successful extravasation and limited survival of early micrometastases. *Am J Pathol* **153**(3): 865–73.

66. Majka, M., Ratajczak, J., et al. (2000). Binding of stromal derived factor-1alpha (SDF-1alpha) to CXCR4 chemokine receptor in normal human megakaryoblasts but not in platelets induces phosphorylation of mitogen-activated protein kinase p42/44 (MAPK), ELK-1 transcription factor and serine/threonine kinase AKT. *Eur J Haematol* **64**(3): 164–72.
67. Mauro, L. and Surmacz E. (2004). IGF-I receptor, cell–cell adhesion, tumour development and progression. *J Mol Histol* **35**(3): 247–53.
68. Mellado, M., Rodriguez-Frade, J. M., et al. (2001). Chemokine signaling and functional responses: the role of receptor dimerization and TK pathway activation. *Annu Rev Immunol* **19**: 397–421.
69. Mitra, P., De, A., et al. (2001). Loss of chemokine SDF-1alpha-mediated CXCR4 signalling and receptor internalization in human hepatoma cell line HepG2. *Cell Signal* **13**(5): 311–9.
70. Moore, B. B., Arenberg, D. A., et al. (1999). Distinct CXC chemokines mediate tumorigenicity of prostate cancer cells. *Am J Pathol* **154**(15): 1503–12.
71. Moore, M. A. (2001). The role of chemoattraction in cancer metastases. *Bioessays* **23**(8): 674–6.
72. Moser, B., L. Barella, et al. (1993). Expression of transcripts for two interleukin 8 receptors in human phagocytes, lymphocytes and melanoma cells. *Biochem J* **294**(Pt 1): 285–92.
73. Muller, A., Homey, B., et al. (2001). Involvement of chemokine receptors in breast cancer metastasis. *Nature* **410**(6824): 50–6.
74. Murakami, T., Maki, W., et al. (2002). Expression of CXC chemokine receptor-4 enhances the pulmonary metastatic potential of murine B16 melanoma cells. *Cancer Res* **62**(24): 7328–34.
75. Murphy, P. M. (2001). Chemokines and the molecular basis of cancer metastasis. *N Engl J Med* **345**(11): 833–5.
76. Musha, H., Ohtani, H., et al. (2005). Selective infiltration of CCR5(+)CXCR3(+) T lymphocytes in human colorectal carcinoma. *Int J Cancer* **116**(6): 949–56.
77. Nagasawa, T., Hirota, S., et al. (1996). Defects of B-cell lymphopoiesis and bone-marrow myelopoiesis in mice lacking the CXC chemokine PBSF/SDF-1. *Nature* **382**(6592): 635–8.
78. Nahta, R., Hortobagyi, G. N., et al. (2003). Growth factor receptors in breast cancer: potential for therapeutic intervention. *Oncologist* **8**(1): 5–17.
79. Negus, R. P., Stamp, G. W., et al. (1997). Quantitative assessment of the leukocyte infiltrate in ovarian cancer and its relationship to the expression of C-C chemokines. *Am J Pathol* **150**(5): 1723–34.
80. Neves, S. R., Ram, P. T., et al. (2002). G protein pathways. *Science* **296**(5573): 1636–9.
81. Nguyen, D. H. and Taub, D. (2002). CXCR4 function requires membrane cholesterol: implications for HIV infection. *J Immunol* **168**(8): 4121–6.
82. Nicolson, G. L. (1993). Cancer progression and growth: relationship of paracrine and autocrine growth mechanisms to organ preference of metastasis. *Exp Cell Res* **204**(2): 171–80.
83. Norgauer, J., Metzner, B., et al. (1996). Expression and growth-promoting function of the IL-8 receptor beta in human melanoma cells. *J Immunol* **156**(3): 1132–37.
84. Ohta, M., Kitadai, Y.,et al. (2002). Monocyte chemoattractant protein-1 expression correlates with macrophage infiltration and tumor vascularity in human esophageal squamous cell carcinomas. *Int J Cancer* **102**(3): 220–4.
85. Owen, J. D., Strieter, R., et al. (1997). Enhanced tumor-forming capacity for immortalized melanocytes expressing melanoma growth stimulatory activity/growth-regulated cytokine beta and gamma proteins. *Int J Cancer* **73**(1): 94–103.
86. Papa, V., Gliozzo, B., et al. (1993). Insulin-like growth factor-I receptors are overexpressed and predict a low risk in human breast cancer. *Cancer Res* **53**(16): 3736–40.

87. Peyrat, J. P. and Bonneterre, J (1992). Type 1 IGF receptor in human breast diseases. *Breast Cancer Res Treat* **22**(1): 59–67.
88. Pike, L. J. (2003). Lipid rafts: bringing order to chaos. *J Lipid Res* **44**(4): 655–67. Epub 2003 Feb 1.
89. Pike, L. J. (2004). Lipid rafts: heterogeneity on the high seas. *Biochem J* **378**(Pt 2): 281–92.
90. Polyak, K. (2001). On the birth of breast cancer. *Biochim Biophys Acta* **1552**(1): 1–13.
91. Pyne, N. J., Waters, C., et al. (2003). Receptor tyrosine kinase-GPCR signal complexes. *Biochem Soc Trans* **31**(Pt 6): 1220–5.
92. Rahmatullah, M. and Robishaw, J. D. (1994). Direct interaction of the alpha and gamma subunits of the G proteins. Purification and analysis by limited proteolysis. *J Biol Chem* **269**(5): 3574–80.
93. Remacle-Bonnet, M., Garrouste, F., et al. (2005). Membrane rafts segregate pro- from anti-apoptotic insulin-like growth factor-I receptor signaling in colon carcinoma cells stimulated by members of the tumor necrosis factor superfamily. *Am J Pathol* **167**(3): 761–73.
94. Robinson, S. C., Scott, K. A., et al. (2002). Chemokine stimulation of monocyte matrix metalloproteinase-9 requires endogenous TNF-alpha. *Eur J Immunol* **32**(2): 404–12.
95. Robledo, M. M., Bartolome, R. A.,et al. (2001). Expression of functional chemokine receptors CXCR3 and CXCR4 on human melanoma cells. *J Biol Chem* **276**(48): 45098–105.
96. Rogers, C. E., Loveday, R. L., et al. (2002). Molecular prognostic indicators in breast cancer. *Eur J Surg Oncol* **28**(5): 467–78.
97. Ruan, W. and Kleinberg, D. L. (1999). Insulin-like growth factor I is essential for terminal end bud formation and ductal morphogenesis during mammary development. *Endocrinology* **140**(11): 5075–81.
98. Sachdev, D., Hartell, J. S., et al. (2004). A dominant negative type I insulin-like growth factor receptor inhibits metastasis of human cancer cells. *J Biol Chem* **279**(6): 5017–24. Epub 2003 Nov 13.
99. Sachdev, D. and Yee, D. (2001). The IGF system and breast cancer. *Endocr Relat Cancer* **8**(3): 197–209.
100. Salcedo, R., Wasserman, K., et al. (1999). Vascular endothelial growth factor and basic fibroblast growth factor induce expression of CXCR4 on human endothelial cells: In vivo neovascularization induced by stromal-derived factor-1alpha. *Am J Pathol* **154**(4): 1125–35.
101. Schadendorf, D., Moller, A., et al. (1993). IL-8 produced by human malignant melanoma cells in vitro is an essential autocrine growth factor. *J Immunol* **151**(5): 2667–75.
102. Schmid, B. C., Rudas, M., et al. (2004). CXCR4 is expressed in ductal carcinoma in situ of the breast and in atypical ductal hyperplasia. *Breast Cancer Res Treat* **84**(3): 247–50.
103. Schneider, M. R., Hoeflich, A., et al. (2000). Interleukin-6 stimulates clonogenic growth of primary and metastatic human colon carcinoma cells. *Cancer Lett* **151**(1): 31–8.
104. Scotton, C. J., Wilson, J. L., et al. (2002). Multiple actions of the chemokine CXCL12 on epithelial tumor cells in human ovarian cancer. *Cancer Res* **62**(20): 5930–8.
105. Simons, K. and Toomre, D. (2000). Lipid rafts and signal transduction. *Nat Rev Mol Cell Biol* **1**(1): 31–9.
106. Singer, C. F., Kubista, E., et al. (2000). Local feedback mechanisms in human breast cancer. *Breast Cancer Res Treat* **63**(2): 95–104.
107. Singh, R. K., Gutman, M., et al. (1994). Expression of interleukin 8 correlates with the metastatic potential of human melanoma cells in nude mice. *Cancer Res* **54**(12): 3242–7.
108. Slamon, D. J., Clark, G. M., et al. (1987). Human breast cancer: correlation of relapse and survival with amplification of the HER-2/neu oncogene. *Science* **235**(4785): 177–82.
109. Slamon, D. J., Godolphin, W., et al. (1989). Studies of the HER-2/neu proto-oncogene in human breast and ovarian cancer. *Science* **244**(4905): 707–12.

110. Smith, M. C., Luker, K. E., et al. (2004). CXCR4 regulates growth of both primary and metastatic breast cancer. *Cancer Res* **64**(23): 8604–12.
111. Soriano, S. F., Hernanz-Falcon, P., et al. (2002). Functional inactivation of CXC chemokine receptor 4-mediated responses through SOCS3 up-regulation. *J Exp Med* **196**(3): 311–21.
112. Speirs, V. and Kerin, M. J. (2000). Prognostic significance of oestrogen receptor beta in breast cancer. *Br J Surg* **87**(4): 405–9.
113. Speirs, V., Parkes, A. T., et al. (1999). Coexpression of estrogen receptor alpha and beta: poor prognostic factors in human breast cancer? *Cancer Res* **59**(3): 525–8.
114. Spiegel, A. M. and Weinstein, L. S. (2004). Inherited diseases involving g proteins and g protein-coupled receptors. *Annu Rev Med* **55**: 27–39.
115. Sporn, M. B. (1996). The war on cancer. *Lancet* **347**(9012): 1377–81.
116. Strieter, R. M., Polverini, P. J., et al. (1995). The functional role of the ELR motif in CXC chemokine-mediated angiogenesis. *J Biol Chem* **270**(45): 27348–57.
117. Surmacz, E. (2000). Function of the IGF-I receptor in breast cancer. *J Mammary Gland Biol Neoplasia* **5**(1): 95–105.
118. Surmacz, E., Guvakova, M. A., et al. (1998). Type I insulin-like growth factor receptor function in breast cancer. *Breast Cancer Res Treat* **47**(3): 255–67.
119. Tachibana, K., Hirota, S., et al. (1998). The chemokine receptor CXCR4 is essential for vascularization of the gastrointestinal tract. *Nature* **393**(6685): 591–4.
120. Takanami, I. (2003). Overexpression of CCR7 mRNA in nonsmall cell lung cancer: correlation with lymph node metastasis. *Int J Cancer* **105**(2): 186–9.
121. Tanaka, T., Z. Bai, et al. (2005). "Chemokines in tumor progression and metastasis." *Cancer Sci* **96**(6): 317–22.
122. Tanimoto, T., Lungu, A. O., et al. (2004). Sphingosine 1-phosphate transactivates the platelet-derived growth factor beta receptor and epidermal growth factor receptor in vascular smooth muscle cells. *Circ Res* **94**(8): 1050–8. Epub 2004 Mar 25.
123. Thelen, M. (2001). Dancing to the tune of chemokines. *Nat Immunol* **2**(2): 129–34.
124. Trentin, L., Cabrelle, A., et al. (2004). Homeostatic chemokines drive migration of malignant B cells in patients with non-Hodgkin lymphomas. *Blood* **104**(2): 502–8. Epub 2004 Mar 4.
125. van Golen, K. L. (2003). Inflammatory breast cancer: relationship between growth factor signaling and motility in aggressive cancers. *Breast Cancer Res* **5**(3): 174–9. Epub 2003 Apr 4.
126. Varney, M. L., Li, A., et al. (2003). Expression of CXCR1 and CXCR2 receptors in malignant melanoma with different metastatic potential and their role in interleukin-8 (CXCL-8)-mediated modulation of metastatic phenotype. *Clin Exp Metastasis* **20**(8): 723–31.
127. Veltri, R. W., Miller, M. C., et al. (1999). Interleukin-8 serum levels in patients with benign prostatic hyperplasia and prostate cancer. *Urology* **53**(1): 139–47.
128. Veronesi, U., Boyle, P., et al. (2005). Breast cancer. *Lancet* **365**(9472): 1727–41.
129. Vicari, A. P. and Caux, C. (2002). "Chemokines in cancer. *Cytokine Growth Factor Rev* **13**(2): 143–54.
130. Walden, P. D., Ruan, W., et al. (1998). Evidence that the mammary fat pad mediates the action of growth hormone in mammary gland development. *Endocrinology* **139**(2): 659–62.
131. Waters, C., Pyne, S., et al. (2004). The role of G-protein coupled receptors and associated proteins in receptor tyrosine kinase signal transduction. *Semin Cell Dev Biol* **15**(3): 309–23.
132. Weiss, L. (1996). Metastatic inefficiency: intravascular and intraperitoneal implantation of cancer cells. *Cancer Treat Res* **82**: 1–11.
133. Wiley, H. E., Gonzalez, E. B., et al. (2001). Expression of CC chemokine receptor-7 and regional lymph node metastasis of B16 murine melanoma. *J Natl Cancer Inst* **93**(21): 1638–43.

134. Youngs, S. J., Ali, S. A., et al. (1997). Chemokines induce migrational responses in human breast carcinoma cell lines. *Int J Cancer* **71**(2): 257–66.
135. Yu, D. and Hung, M. C. (2000). Overexpression of ErbB2 in cancer and ErbB2-targeting strategies. *Oncogene* **19**(53): 6115–21.
136. Zhou, Y., Larsen, P. H., et al. (2002). CXCR4 is a major chemokine receptor on glioma cells and mediates their survival. *J Biol Chem* **277**(51): 49481–7.
137. Zlotnik, A. and Yoshie, O., (2000). Chemokines: a new classification system and their role in immunity. *Immunity* **12**(2): 121–7.
138. Zou, Y. R., Kottmann, A. H., et al. (1998). Function of the chemokine receptor CXCR4 in haematopoiesis and in cerebellar development. *Nature* **393**(6685): 595–9.
139. Zwick, E., Bange, J., et al. (2001). Receptor tyrosine kinase signalling as a target for cancer intervention strategies. *Endocr Relat Cancer* **8**(3): 161–73.

CXCR4 and Cancer

Bungo Furusato and Johng S. Rhim

Abstract The chemokine receptor CXCR4 belongs to the large superfamily of G-protein-coupled receptors, and is directly involved in a number of biological processes including organogenesis, hematopoiesis, and immunity. Recent evidence has highlighted the role of CXCR4 in a variety of diseases including cancer and WHIM syndrome. Expression of CXCR4 in cancer metastasis appears to be due to dysregulation of the receptor leading to enhanced signaling. CXCR4 was also found to be a prognostic marker in various types of cancer including leukemia and breast cancer. These observations reveal that CXCR4 is an important molecule involved in several aspects of cancer progression. The SDF-1-CXCR4 axis is also involved in normal stem cell homing. Interestingly, cancer stem cells also express CXCR4 suggesting that the SDF-1-CXCR4 axis directs their trafficking/metastasis to organs that highly express SDF-1 such as the lymph nodes, lungs, liver, and bones. Here, we review what is currently known regarding the regulation of CXCR4 and how dysregulation contributes to disease progression.

The Chemokine Receptor CXCR4 and Cancer

The human chemokine system currently includes more than 40 chemokines and 18 chemokine receptors (Table 1). Chemokine receptors are defined by their ability to induce directional migration of cells toward a gradient of a chemotactic cytokine (chemotaxis). Chemokine receptors belong to a family of 7 transmembrane domain, G-protein-coupled cell surface receptors (GPCR) and the ligands are classified into four groups (CXC, CC, C, and CX_3C) based on the position of the first two cysteines [1, 2]. Chemokine receptors are present on many different cell types. Initially, these receptors were identified on

J.S. Rhim (✉)
Department of Surgery, Center for Prostate Disease Research, Uniformed Service
University of the Health Science, Bethesda, MD 20814, USA
e-mail: jrhim@verizon.net

A.M. Fulton (ed.), *Chemokine Receptors in Cancer*, Cancer Drug Discovery
and Development, DOI 10.1007/978-1-60327-267-4_2,
© Humana Press, a part of Springer Science+Business Media, LLC 2009

Table 1 Chemokine receptors and ligands

Recepter	Ligand
CXC Chemokine	
CXCR1	GCP-2/CXCL6, IL-8/CXCL8
CXCR2	GROα,β,γ/CXCL1,2,3, ENA-78/CXCL5, GCP-2/CXCL6, IL-8/CXCL8
CXCR3	MIG/CXCL9, IP-10/CXCL10, I-TAC/CXCL11, BLC/CXCL 13, SLC/CCL21
CXCR4	SDF-1/CXCL12
CXCR5	CXCL13/BLC
CXCR6	CXCL16
CC Chemokine	
CCR1	MIP-1α/CCL3, RANTES/CCL5, MCP-3/CCL7, MCP-2/CCL8, LD78β/CCL3L1, HCC-1/CCL14, Lkn-1/CCL15, LEC/CCL16, MPIF-1/CCL23
CCR2	MCP-1/CCL2, MCP-2/CCL8, MCP-3/CCL7, MCP-4/CCL13, LEC/CCL16
CCR3	RANTES/CCL5, MCP-2/CCL8, MCP-3/CCL7, MCP-4/CCL13, eotaxin-1,2,3/CCL11, 24, 26, LD78β/CCL3L1, Lkn-1/CCL15, MEC/CCL28
CCR4	TARC/CCL17, MDC/CCL22
CCR5	MIP-1α/CCL3, MIP-1β/CCL4, RANTES/CCL5, MCP-2/CCL8, LD78β/CCL3L1, LEC/CCL16
CCR6	LARC/CCL20, β-defensin
CCR7	ELC/CCL19, SLC/CCL21
CCR8	I-309/CCL1
CCR9	TECK/CCL25
CCR10	ILC/CCL27, MEC/CCL28
C Chemokine	
XCR1	SCM-1/XCL1,2
CX$_3$C Chemokine	
CX$_3$CR1	fractalkine/CX$_3$CL1

leukocytes, where they were found to play an important role in the "homing" of such cells to sites of inflammation [3].

During the past several years, other types of cells (nonhematopoietic) also have been found to express receptors for various chemokines present in their distinct tissue microenvironments. The interactions between such receptors and their respective chemokines are thought to help coordinate the trafficking and organization of cells within various tissue compartments [4, 5].

CXCR4 is one of the most studied chemokine receptors, primarily due to its role as a coreceptor for HIV entry [6] as well as its ability to mediate the metastasis of a variety of cancers including prostate cancer [7–11].

CXCR4 is a 352 amino acid rhodopsin-like GPCR that selectively binds the CXC chemokine stromal cell-derived factor 1 (SDF-1), also known as CXCL12 [1, 12].

In animal models, the lack of either SDF-1 or CXCR4 exhibits an almost identical phenotype of late gestational lethality and defects in B cell lymphopoiesis, bone marrow colonization, and cardiac septum formation [13, 14]. These studies indicated that CXCR4 is essential for development, hematopoiesis, organogenesis, and vascularization [13–19], in addition to functioning as a classical chemokine receptor in adults [5, 19].

There is growing evidence that CXCR4 functions not only in cancer metastasis but it also seems to be involved in the "cancer stem cell" process. The physiologic mechanisms of tissue-specific recruitment features (the "homing" system for normal tissue replacement) also seem functional in cancer cells.

This review will focus on the role of CXCR4 in cancer, particularly in the putative cancer stem cell. We will discuss what is known about the factors involved in receptor expression and regulation, how dysregulation of these pathways may contribute to disease progression, and the potential options for targeted therapy.

Concept of Cancer Stem Cells

The growing evidence shows that quiescent tissue-committed stem cells (TCSCs), cells that are closely related to the development of each organ, may be the origin of cancer development. The concept of cancer stem cells has been postulated by several investigators since it was initially documented by experiments in human leukemias [20]. Stem cells are long-living cells and thus become a potential target for cell damage; they will be subjected to accumulating mutations, which are crucial for the initiation and progression of cancer. Several studies have shown that mutations that occur in normal stem cells can lead to their malignant transformation and tumor initiation [21–23].

A recent study shows that the stem cell origin of cancer was demonstrated in several solid tumors such as brain, breast, and prostate cancers [24–26]. They also are thought to be "tough guys" in response to chemotherapy. Since cancer stem cells are similar to normal stem cells, when they exist in a quiescent state they are relatively resistant to most anticancer drugs which target only dividing cells. Cancer stem cells only represent a subpopulation of a growing tumor. They are capable of initiating metastasis and they regroup (or function as "seeds") to form new tumors after unsuccessful treatment.

The bottom line is that CXCR4 is expressed in the normal stem cells of different organs/tissues. This may help to explain why some tumors express CXCR4, and why we believe these malignant cells may derive from CXCR4 expressing normal stem cells (Table 2).

Table 2 Examples of tumors expressing CXCR4 that may derive from the normal stem cells which express CXCR4 (Adapted From Ref #9)

Normal cells	Corresponding tumor
Prostate gland epithelial stem cells	Prostate cancer
Hematopoietic stem cells	Leukemias
Neural stem cells	Brain tumors
Mammary gland epithelial stem cells	Breast cancer
Skeletal muscle satellite cells	Rhabdomyosarcoma
Neuroectodermal stem cells	Neuroblastoma
Renal tubular epithelial stem cells	Wilms' tumor
Retina pigment epithelial stem cells	Retinoblastoma
Liver oval stem cells	Hepatoblastoma
Ovarian epithelial stem cells	Ovarian cancer
Cervical epithelial stem cells	Cervical cancer

The Role of CXCR4-SDF-1 Axis Involved in Mobilization, Trafficking, and Homing of Cancer Stem Cells

The SDF-1–CXCR4 axis may influence the biology of tumors. It is believed that the organs that express high SDF-1 (e.g., lymph nodes, lungs, liver, or bones) may direct the metastasis of CXCR4-expressing tumor cells.

Supporting this hypothesis, it has been reported that several cancers expressing CXCR4 (e.g., breast, ovarian, and prostate cancers, rhabdomyosarcoma, and neuroblastoma) metastasize to the bones through the bloodstream in an SDF-1-dependent manner [11, 25, 27–32]. The role of the SDF-1–CXCR4 axis in regulating the trafficking/homing of tumor cell metastasis seems to share some of the molecular mechanisms involved in normal stem cell processes. Seen from this perspective, the mobilization, trafficking, and homing of both cancer and normal stem cells seem to involve multistep processes as described in several studies [9, 33–35] (Fig. 1).

CXCR4 Receptor Expression, Regulation, and Pathway

Interestingly, CXCR4 is expressed in a variety of cancers but its expression in the adjacent normal tissue is rare [11, 27, 36]. This may result from changes that occur within the vasculature or the O_2-carrying capacity of cells, leading to hypoxic conditions during tumor progression [37]. Hypoxia induces the activation of hypoxia inducible factor 1 (HIF-1) which may also promote expression of a number of target genes including CXCR4 [37–40].

This function of HIF-1 was discovered in studies of the tumor suppressor gene, von Hippel Lindau (VHL). Inactivating mutations of VHL, which

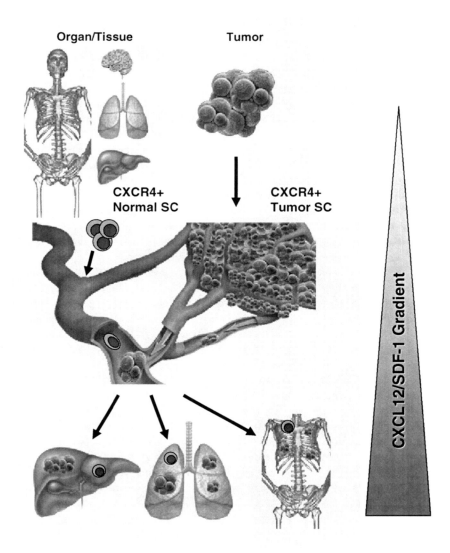

Fig. 1 The role of the SDF-1–CXCR4 axis in migration/circulation of normal stem cells and metastasis of cancer stem cells. Migration of normal stem cells and metastasis of malignant stem cells is a multistep process in which cells (I) leave their stem cell niches (normal stem cells) or primary tumor (cancer stem cells) and enter circulation, (II) arrive at the site of homing (normal stem cells) or metastasis (malignant stem cells) via the peripheral blood or lymph, (III) adhere to the endothelium, (IV) invade tissues, and proliferate and expand at a location that provides a supportive environment for them. We hypothesize that CXCL12/SDF-1 plays a crucial role in this process, chemoattracting CXCR4 + normal or tumor stem cells. Abbreviations: SC stem cell, SDF stromal-derived factor. (Modified from Kucia M., Reca R., Miekus K., et al. (2005) Trafficking of normal stem cells and metastasis of cancer stem cells involve similar mechanisms: Pivotal role of the SDF-1-CXCR4 axis. *Stem Cells*, **23**. 879–94.)

normally targets HIF-1 for degradation, account for the increased CXCR4 expression in renal cell carcinomas [38–40].

The vascular endothelial growth factor (VEGF) [41] and/or activation of nuclear factor kappa B (NF-κB) [42] also have the ability to increase CXCR4 expression specifically during cancer progression. These genes enhance CXCR4 expression in breast cancer, promoting invasion and metastasis.

Further, it has been shown that oncoproteins also induce CXCR4 expression. These are known as PAX3–FKHR [31, 43] and RET/PTC [44]. The PAX3–FKHR fusion leads to enhanced migration and adhesion of rhabdomyosarcoma cells [31], while RET/PTC-induced expression enhanced the transforming ability of breast cancer cells [44].

Tumor progression, especially in tumor metastasis, is also affected by CXCR4–SDF-1 signaling through the induction of tumor-associated integrin activation and signaling [45]. CXCR4 also stimulates the production of matrix metalloproteases [46–49]. SDF signaling is also able to enhance integrin activity [50–52], enhancing cell adhesion under flow conditions.

If CXCR4 truly mediates metastasis, when tumors enter the blood or lymphatic systems, they would preferentially migrate and adhere to areas with high expression of SDF-1. Breast cancer follows this pattern of metastasis, migrating to lymph nodes, lung, liver, and bone marrow, all of which have high expression of SDF-1 [30, 53]. In vivo, neutralizing antibodies to CXCR4 [30], or silencing CXCR3 by siRNA [54, 55] inhibited the metastasis and growth of breast cancer cells.

Other cancers, such as small cell lung cancer, thyroid, neuroblastoma, hematological, and hepatic malignancies also metastasize to areas with high SDF-1 expression [28, 56–59]. Previous studies have suggested that expression of CXCR4 in hepatocellular carcinoma correlates with local tumor progression, lymphatic and distant metastasis, as well as negatively impacting the 3-year survival rate of these patients [59].

Epigenetic mechanisms that negatively regulate the expression of SDF or CXCR4 may be necessary for tumor metastasis. One example is DNA methylation, a modification typically associated with inactivation of tumor suppressors, and it has been shown that methylation of the SDF promoter in colonic epithelium promotes metastasis of these tumors [60, 61]. Also, the CXCR4 promoter was found to be regulated by DNA methylation in pancreatic cancer, which shows decreasing mRNA and protein levels [62].

Further, the CXCR4 COOH-terminal domain also seems to play a major role in regulating receptors, including epithelial-to-mesenchymal transition (EMT) [63, 64]. Previous studies suggest the C-terminal truncation mutations in the chemokine receptor CXCR4 in warts, hypogammaglobulinemia, immunodeficiency, and myelokathexis (WHIM) syndrome are the first examples of aberrant chemokine receptor function causing human disease [63]. It also has been shown that expression of C-tail truncated mutant of CXCR4 in MCF-7 mammary carcinoma cells exhibits a higher growth rate and alters morphology as indicated by EMT [64].

Taken together, CXCR4 seems to control many diverse processes, from development to cancer metastasis. A large amount of work has been generated in delineating potential pathways that mediate specific effects (e.g., leading to metastasis); however, a detailed receptor regulation process has not been well established yet. Understanding the precise mechanisms regulating CXCR4 function at the receptor level may provide new insight into attractive therapeutic targets in this pathway.

Conclusion and Future Directions

The concept of chemokines influencing the metastatic destination is beginning to be understood. The pictures of chemokine receptors expressed by cancer stem cells seem to represent an important aspect of tumorigenesis and metastasis. The expression of CXCR4 in cancer stem cells is likely to be involved in the organ-specific metastasis, that is, prostate cancer metastasizing to the bone. However, even if the overall findings and hypothesis are correct, in the real world, any such therapeutic method (e.g., a CXCR4 antagonist for a prostate cancer patient with bone metastasis) is unlikely to be used alone, but rather used in combination with established chemotherapy protocols.

From the basic science aspect, there is a lot to learn about CXCR4 and its association with cancers (Table 3). CXCR4 involvement in cancer metastasis mechanisms suggests that CXCR4 antagonism may be a potential option for tackling cancer metastasis [65]. Transfecting CXCR4 into a tumor cell greatly enhances its metastatic potential [140]. Therefore, instead of trying to antagonize this receptor, it may be better to modulate CXCR4 expression in tumor cells to prevent metastasis.

Targeting cancer stem cells may offer improvements in therapy in addition to targeting CXCR4, and future studies are likely to include the identification of cancer stem cell specific surface markers for antibody therapy, elucidation of cancer stem cell specific pathways that can be pharmacologically targeted, and evaluation of agents that promote the differentiation of cancer stem cells into progenitors that do not self-renew.

While the role of CXCR4 and cancer stem cells present exciting clinical implications, its widespread acceptance and application to the practice of medicine has yet to occur.

We anticipate that the findings described in this chapter will be identified in additional tumor types, and knowledge of the detailed biology and clinical significance of this experimentally defined population will provide further support to the concept.

Ultimately, focusing research efforts on the role of CXCR4 and cancer stem cell may drive important advances in our understanding of cancer biology and developing potential cures for these devastating diseases.

Table 3 CXCR4 expression in various cancers

Cancer expressing CXCR4	Reference number
Colon Cancer	[66–68]
Breast Cancer	[69–73]
Lung Cancer	[74–80]
Ovarian Cancer	[81–86]
Prostate Cancer	[87–92]
Kidney Cancer	[93–97]
Brain Cancer	[98, 100–105]
Thyroid Cancer	[44, 57, 106, 107]
Liver Cancer	[59]
Pancreatic Cancer	[108–113]
Esophageal Cancer	[114–116]
Cervical Cancer	[117–119]
Oral Cancer	[120–123]
Melanoma	[124–132]
Leukemia	[133–139]

References

1. Murphy P. M., Baggiolini M., Charo I. F., et al.(2000) International union of pharmacology. XXII. Nomenclature for chemokine receptors.*Pharmacol Rev*, **52**, 145–76.
2. Zlotnik A and Yoshie O. (2000) Chemokines: A new classification system and their role in immunity. *Immunity*, **12**, 121–7.
3. Loetscher P., Moser B., and Baggiolini M. (2000) Chemokines and their receptors in lymphocyte traffic and HIV infection. *Adv Immunol*, **74**, 127–180.
4. Baggiolini M. (1998) Chemokines and leukocyte traffic. *Nature*, **392**, 565–8.
5. Moser B. and Loetscher P. (2001) Lymphocyte traffic control by chemokines. *Nat Immunol.*, **2**, 123–8.
6. Feng Y., Broder C. C., Kennedy P. E., and Berger E. A. (1996. HIV-1 entry cofactor: Functional cDNA cloning of a seven-transmembrane, G protein-coupled receptor. *Science*, **272**, 872–7.
7. Zlotnik A. (2006) Involvement of chemokine receptors in organ-specific metastasis. *Contrib Microbiol.*, **13**, 191–9.
8. Burger J. A.and Kipps T.J. (2006) CXCR4: a key receptor in the crosstalk between tumor cells and their microenvironment. *Blood*, **107**, 1761–7.
9. Kucia M., Reca R., Miekus K., et al. (2005) Trafficking of normal stem cells and metastasis of cancer stem cells involve similar mechanisms: Pivotal role of the SDF-1-CXCR4 axis. *Stem Cells*, **23**. 879–94.
10. Zlotnik A. (2006) Chemokines and cancer. *Int J Cancer.*, **119**, 2026–9.
11. Sun Y. X., Wang J., Shelburne C. E., et al. (2003). Expression of CXCR4 and CXCL12 (SDF-1) in human prostate cancers (PCa) in vivo. *J Cell Biochem.*, **89**, 462–73.
12. Fredriksson R., Lagerström M.C., Lundin L.G., and Schiöth HB (2003) The G-protein-coupled receptors in the human genome form five main families. Phylogenetic analysis, paralogon groups, and fingerprints. *Mol Pharmacol.*, **63**, 1256–72.
13. Nagasawa T., Hirota S., Tachibana K., et al. (1996) Defects of B-cell lymphopoiesis and bone-marrowmyelopoiesis in mice lacking the CXC chemokine PBSF/SDF-1. *Nature*, **382**, 635–8.
14. Zou Y. R., Kottmann A.H., Kuroda M., et al. (1998) Function of the chemokine receptor CXCR4 in haematopoiesis and in cerebellar development. *Nature*, **393**, 595–9.

15. Ma Q., Jones D., Borghesani P. R., Segal R. A., et al. (1998) Impaired B-lymphopoiesis, myelopoiesis, and derailed cerebellar neuron migration in CXCR4- and SDF-1-deficient mice. *Proc Natl Acad Sci U S A.*, **95**, 9448–53.
16. McGrath K. E., Koniski A. D., Maltby K. M., et al. (1999) Embryonic expression and function of the chemokine SDF-1 and its receptor, CXCR4. *Dev Biol.*, **213**, 442–56.
17. Nagasawa T., Tachibana K., and Kishimoto T. (1998) A novel CXC chemokine PBSF/SDF-1 and its receptor CXCR4: their functions in development, hematopoiesis and HIV infection. *Semin Immunol.*, **10**, 179–85.
18. Tachibana K., Hirota S., Iizasa H., et al. (1998) The chemokine receptor CXCR4 is essential for vascularization of the gastrointestinal tract. *Nature.*, **393**, 591–4.
19. Murphy P. M. (1994) The molecular biology of leukocyte chemoattractant receptors. *Annu Rev Immunol.*, **12**, 593–633.
20. Lapidot T., Pflumio F., Doedens M., et al.(1992) Cytokine stimulation of multilineagehematopoiesis from immature human cells engrafted in SCID mice. *Science*, **255**, 1137–41.
21. Tavor S., Petit I., Porozov S., et al. (2004) CXCR4 regulates migration and development of human acute myelogenous leukemia stem cells in transplanted NOD/SCID mice. *Cancer Res.*, **64**, 2817–24.
22. Pardal R., Clarke M. F., and Morrison S.J. (2003) Applying the principles of stem-cell biology to cancer. *Nat Rev Cancer.*, **3**, 895–902.
23. Reya T., Morrison S. J., Clarke M. F., and Weissman I. L. (2001). Stem cells, cancer, and cancer stem cells. *Nature.* **414**, 105–11.
24. Singh S. K , Hawkins C., Clarke I. D., et al. (2004) Identification of human brain tumour initiating cells. *Nature* **432**, 396–401.
25. Dontu G., Al-Hajj M., Abdallah W. M., et al. (2003) Stem cells in normal breast development and breast cancer. *Cell Prolif.* **36**, 59–72.
26. Collins A. T. and Maitland N. J. (2006) Prostate cancer stem cells. *Eur J Cancer.*, **42**, 1213–8.
27. Müller A., Homey B., Soto H., et al. (2001) Involvement of chemokine receptors in breast cancer metastasis. *Nature,* **410**, 50–6.
28. Geminder H., Sagi-Assif O., Goldberg L., et al. (2001) A possible role for CXCR4 and its ligand, the CXC chemokinestromal cell-derived factor-1, in the development of bone marrow metastases in neuroblastoma. *J Immunol.*, **167**, 4747–57.
29. Porcile C., Bajetto A., Barbero S., et al. (2004) CXCR4 activation induces epidermal growth factor receptor transactivation in an ovarian cancer cell line. *Ann N Y Acad Sci.*, **1030**, 162–9.
30. Hall J. M. and Korach K. S. (2003) Stromal cell-derived factor 1, a novel target of estrogen receptor action, mediates the mitogenic effects of estradiol in ovarian and breast cancer cells. *Mol Endocrinol.*, **17**, 792–803.
31. Libura J., Drukala J., Majka M., et al. (2002) CXCR4-SDF-1 signaling is active in rhabdomyosarcoma cells and regulates locomotion, chemotaxis, and adhesion. *Blood*, **100**, 2597–606.
32. Jankowski K., Kucia M., Wysoczynski M., et al. (2003) Both hepatocyte growth factor (HGF) and stromal-derived factor-1 regulate the metastatic behavior of human rhabdomyosarcoma cells, but only HGF enhances their resistance to radiochemotherapy. *Cancer Res.*, **63**, 7926–35.
33. Petit I, Szyper-Kravitz M., Nagler A., Lahav M., et al. (2002) G-CSF induces stem cell mobilization by decreasing bone marrow SDF-1 and up-regulating CXCR4. *Nat Immunol.*, **3**, 687–94.
34. Lapidot T and Petit I. (2002) Current understanding of stem cell mobilization: the roles of chemokines, proteolytic enzymes, adhesion molecules, cytokines, and stromal cells. *Exp Hematol.*, **30**, 973–81.
35. Hattori K., Heissig B., Tashiro K., et al. (2001) Plasma elevation of stromal cell-derived factor-1 induces mobilization of mature and immature hematopoietic progenitor and stem cells. *Blood*, 97:3354–60.

36. Scotton C. J., Wilson J. L., Milliken D., et al (2001) Epithelial cancer cell migration: A role for chemokine receptors? *Cancer Res.*, **61**, 4961–5.
37. Hirota K. and Semenza G. L. (2006) Regulation of angiogenesis by hypoxia-inducible factor 1. *Crit Rev Oncol Hematol.*, 59, 15–26.
38. Schioppa T., Uranchimeg B., Saccani A., et al. (2003) Regulation of the chemokine receptor CXCR4 by hypoxia. *J Exp Med.*, **198**, 1391–402.
39. Staller P., Sulitkova J., Lisztwan J., et al. (2003) Chemokine receptor CXCR4 down-regulated by von Hippel-Lindautumour suppressor pVHL. *Nature*, **425**, 307–11.
40. Zagzag D., Krishnamachary B., Yee H., et al.(2005) Stromal cell-derived factor-1alpha and CXCR4 expression in hemangioblastoma and clear cell-renal cell carcinoma: von Hippel-Lindau loss-of-function induces expression of a ligand and its receptor. *Cancer Res.*, **65**, 6178–88.
41. Bachelder R. E., Wendt M. A., and Mercurio A. M. (2002) Vascular endothelial growth factor promotes breast carcinoma invasion in an autocrine manner by regulating the chemokine receptor CXCR4. *Cancer Res.* 62, 7203–6.
42. Helbig G., Christopherson K. W. 2nd, Bhat-Nakshatri P., et al. (2003) NF-kappaB promotes breast cancer cell migration and metastasis by inducing the expression of the chemokine receptor CXCR4. *J Biol Chem.*, **278**, 21631–8.
43. Tomescu O., Xia S. J., Strzlecki D., et al. (2004) Inducible short-term and stable long-term cell culture systems reveal that the PAX3-FKHR fusion oncoprotein regulates CXCR4, PAX3, and PAX7 expression. *Lab Invest.*, **84**, 1060–70.
44. Castellone M. D., Guarino V., De Falco V., et al. (2004) Functional expression of the CXCR4 chemokine receptor is induced by RET/PTC oncogenes and is a common event in human papillary thyroid carcinomas. *Oncogene*, **23**, 5958–67.
45. Hartmann T. N., Burger J. A., Glodek A., et al. (2005) CXCR4 chemokine receptor and integrin signaling co-operate in mediating adhesion and chemoresistance in small cell lung cancer (SCLC) cells. *Oncogene,*, 4462–71.
46. Fernandis A. Z., Prasad A., Band H., et al. (2004) Regulation of CXCR4-mediated chemotaxis and chemoinvasion of breast cancer cells. *Oncogene*, **23**, 157–67.
47. Janowska-Wieczorek A., Marquez L. A., Dobrowsky A., et al. (2000) Differential MMP and TIMP production by human marrow and peripheral blood CD34(+) cells in response to chemokines. *Exp Hematol.*, **28**, 1274–85.
48. Samara G. J., Lawrence D. M., Chiarelli C. J., et al. (2004) CXCR4-mediated adhesion and MMP-9 secretion in head and neck squamous cell carcinoma. *Cancer Lett.*, **214**, 231–41.
49. Spiegel A., Kollet O., Peled A., et al. (2004) Unique SDF-1-induced activation of human precursor-B all cells as a result of altered CXCR4 expression and signaling. *Blood*, **103**, 2900–7.
50. Campbell J.J., Hedrick J., Zlotnik A., et al. (1998) Chemokines and the arrest of lymphocytes rolling under flow conditions. *Science.*, **279**, 381–4.
51. Glodek A. M., Honczarenko M., Le Y., et al. (2003) Sustained activation of cell adhesion is a differentially regulated process in B lymphopoiesis. *J Exp Med.*, **197**, 461–73.
52. Wright N., Hidalgo A., Rodríguez-Frade J. M., et al. (2002) The chemokinestromal cell-derived factor-1 alpha modulates alpha 4 beta 7 integrin-mediated lymphocyte adhesion to mucosal addressin cell adhesion molecule-1 and fibronectin. *J Immunol.*, **168**, 5268–77.
53. Allinen M., Beroukhim R., Cai L., et al. (2004) Molecular characterization of the tumor microenvironment in breast cancer. *Cancer Cell*, **6**, 17–32.
54. Lapteva N., Yang A. G., Sanders D. E., et al. (2005) CXCR4 knockdown by small interfering RNA abrogates breast tumor growth in vivo. *Cancer Gene Ther.*, **12**, 84–9.
55. Liang Z., Yoon Y., Votaw J., et al. (2005) Silencing of CXCR4 blocks breast cancer metastasis. *Cancer Res.*, **65**, 967–71.
56. Burger M., Glodek A., Hartmann T., et al. (2003) Functional expression of CXCR4 (CD184) on small-cell lung cancer cells mediates migration, integrin activation, and adhesion to stromal cells. *Oncogene.*, **22**, 8093–101.

57. Hwang J. H., Hwang J. H., Chung H. K., et al. (2003) CXC chemokine receptor 4 expression and function in human anaplastic thyroid cancer cells. *J Clin Endocrinol Metab.*, **88**, 408–16.
58. Kijima T., Maulik G., Ma P. C., et al. (2002) Regulation of cellular proliferation, cytoskeletal function, and signal transduction through CXCR4 and c-Kit in small cell lung cancer cells. *Cancer Res.*, **62**, 6304–11.
59. Schimanski C. C., Bahre R., Gockel I., et al. (2006) Dissemination of hepatocellular carcinoma is mediated via chemokine receptor CXCR4. *Br J Cancer.*, **95**, 210–7.
60. Jones P. A. and Baylin S. B. (2002) The fundamental role of epigenetic events in cancer. *Nat Rev Genet.* **3**, 415–28.
61. Wendt M. K., Johanesen P. A., Kang-Decker N., et al.(2006) Silencing of epithelial CXCL12 expression by DNA hypermethylation promotes colonic carcinoma metastasis. ., **25**, 4986–97.
62. Sato N., Matsubayashi H., Fukushima N., and Goggins M. (2005) The chemokine receptor CXCR4 is regulated by DNA methylation in pancreatic cancer. *Cancer Biol Ther.*, **4**, 70–6.
63. Hernandez P. A., Gorlin R. J., Lukens J. N., et al. (2003) Mutations in the chemokine receptor gene CXCR4 are associated with WHIM syndrome, a combined immunodeficiency disease. *Nat Genet.*, **34**, 70–4.
64. Ueda Y., Neel N. F., Schutyser E., et al. (2006) Deletion of the COOH-terminal domain of CXC chemokine receptor 4 leads to the down-regulation of cell-to-cell contact, enhanced motility and proliferation in breast carcinoma cells. *Cancer Res.*, **66**, 5665–75.
65. Zhang W. B., Navenot J. M., Haribabu B., et al. (2002) A point mutation that confers constitutive activity to CXCR4 reveals that T140 is an inverse agonist and that AMD3100 and ALX40–4C are weak partial agonists. *J Biol Chem.*, **277**, 24515–21.
66. Ottaiano A., di Palma A., Napolitano M., et al. (2005) Inhibitory effects of anti-CXCR4 antibodies on human colon cancer cells. *Cancer Immunol Immunother.*, **54**, 781–91.
67. Zeelenberg I. S., Ruuls-Van Stalle L., and Roos E. (2003) The chemokine receptor CXCR4 is required for outgrowth of colon carcinoma micrometastases. *Cancer Ries.*, **63**, 3833–9.
68. Mitra P., Shibuta K., Mathai J., et al. (1999). CXCR4 mRNA expression in colon, esophageal and gastric cancers and hepatitis C infected liver. *Int J Oncol.*, **14**, 917–25.
69. Chen Y., Stamatoyannopoulos G., and Song C. Z. (2003) Down-regulation of CXCR4 by inducible small interfering RNA inhibits breast cancer cell invasion in vitro. *Cancer Res.*, **63**, 4801–4.
70. Benovic J. L. and Marchese A. (2004) A new key in breast cancer metastasis. *Cancer Cell.*, **6**, 429–30.
71. Epstein R. J. (2004) The CXCL12-CXCR4 chemotactic pathway as a target of adjuvant breast cancer therapies. *Nat Rev Cancer.*, **4**, 901–9.
72. Cabioglu N., Summy J., Miller C., et al. (2005) CXCL-12/stromal cell-derived factor-1alpha transactivates HER2-neu in breast cancer cells by a novel pathway involving Src kinase activation. *Cancer Res.*, **65**, 6493–7.
73. Orimo A., Gupta P. B., Sgroi D. C., et al. (2005) Stromal fibroblasts present in invasive human breast carcinomas promote tumor growth and angiogenesis through elevated SDF-1/CXCL12 secretion. *Cell.* **121**, 335–48.
74. Huang Y. C., Hsiao Y. C., Chen Y. J., et al. (2007) Stromal cell-derived factor-1 enhances motility and integrin up-regulation through CXCR4, ERK and NF-kappaB-dependent pathway in human lung cancer cells. *Biochem Pharmacol.*, **74**, 1702–12.
75. Phillips R. J., Burdick M. D., Lutz M., et al. (2003). The stromal derived factor-1/ CXCL12-CXC chemokine receptor 4 biological axis in non-small cell lung cancer metastases. *Am J Respir Crit Care Med.*, **167**, 1676–86.
76. Oonakahara K., Matsuyama W., Higashimoto I., et al. (2004) Stromal-derived factor-1alpha/CXCL12-CXCR 4 axis is involved in the dissemination of NSCLC cells into pleural space. *Am J Respir Cell Mol Biol.*, 3b0, 671–7.

77. Spano J. P., Andre F., Morat L., et al. (2004) Chemokine receptor CXCR4 and early-stage non-small cell lung cancer: Pattern of expression and correlation with outcome. *Ann Oncol.*, **15**, 613–7.
78. Belperio J. A., Phillips R. J., Burdick M. D., et al.(2004) The SDF-1/CXCL 12/CXCR4 biological axis in non-small cell lung cancer metastases. *Chest*, **125**, 156S.
79. Hartmann T. N., Burger M., and Burger J. A. (2004) The role of adhesion molecules and chemokine receptor CXCR4 (CD184) in small cell lung cancer. *J Biol Regul Homeost Agents.*, **18**, 126–30.
80. Phillips R. J., Mestas J., Gharaee-Kermani M., et al. (2005) Epidermal growth factor and hypoxia-induced expression of CXC chemokine receptor 4 on non-small cell lung cancer cells is regulated by the phosphatidylinositol 3-kinase/PTEN/AKT/mammalian target of rapamycin signaling pathway and activation of hypoxia inducible factor-1alpha. *J Biol Chem.*, **280**, 22473–81.
81. Kajiyama H., Shibata K., Terauchi M., et al. (2008) Involvement of SDF-1alpha/CXCR4 axis in the enhanced peritoneal metastasis of epithelial ovarian carcinoma. *Int J Cancer.*, **122**, 91–9.
82. Furuya M., Suyama T., Usui H., et al. (2007) Up-regulation of CXC chemokines and their receptors: implications for proinflammatory microenvironments of ovarian carcinomas and endometriosis. *Hum Pathol.*, **38**, 1676–87.
83. Oda Y., Ohishi Y., Basaki Y., et al. (2007) Prognostic implications of the nuclear localization of Y-box-binding protein-1 and CXCR4 expression in ovarian cancer: their correlation with activated Akt, LRP/MVP and P-glycoprotein expression. *Cancer Sci.*, **98**, 1020–6.
84. Kulbe H., Hagemann T., Szlosarek P. W., et al. (2005) The inflammatory cytokine tumor necrosis factor-alpha regulates chemokine receptor expression on ovarian cancer cells. *Cancer Res.*, **65**, 10355–62.
85. Kryczek I., Lange A., Mottram P., et al. (2005) CXCL12 and vascular endothelial growth factor synergistically induce neoangiogenesis in human ovarian cancers. *Cancer Res.*, **65**, 465–72.
86. Scotton C. J., Wilson J. L., Scott K., et al. (2002) Multiple actions of the chemokine CXCL12 on epithelial tumor cells in human ovarian cancer. *Cancer Res.*, **62**, 5930–8.
87. Taichman R. S., Cooper C., Keller E. T., et al. (2002) Use of the stromal cell-derived factor-1/CXCR4 pathway in prostate cancer metastasis to bone. *Cancer Res.*, **62**, 1832–7.
88. Chinni S. R., Sivalogan S., Dong Z., et al. (2006) CXCL12/CXCR4 signaling activates Akt-1 and MMP-9 expression in prostate cancer cells: The role of bone microenvironment-associated CXCL12. *Prostate*, **66**, 32–48.
89. Miwa S., Mizokami A., Keller E. T., et al. (2005) The bisphosphonate YM529 inhibits osteolytic and osteoblastic changes and CXCR-4-induced invasion in prostate cancer. *Cancer Res.*, **65**, 8818–25.
90. Engl T., Relja B., Marian D., et al. (2006) CXCR4 chemokine receptor mediates prostate tumor cell adhesion through alpha5 and beta3 integrins. *Neoplasia.* **8**, 290–301.
91. Miki J., Furusato B., Li H., et al. (2007) Identification of putative stem cell markers, CD133 and CXCR4, in hTERT-immortalized primary nonmalignant and malignant tumor-derived human prostate epithelial cell lines and in prostate cancer specimens. *Cancer Res.*, **67**, 3153–61.
92. Hirata H., Hinoda Y., Kikuno N., et al. (2007) CXCL12 G801A polymorphism is a risk factor for sporadic prostate cancer susceptibility. *Clin Cancer Res.*, **13**, 5056–62.
93. Gerritsen M. E., Peale F. V. Jr, and Wu T. (2002) Gene expression profiling in silico: Relative expression of candidate angiogenesis associated genes in renal cell carcinomas. *Exp Nephrol.*, 10, 114–9.
94. Schrader A. J., Lechner O., Templin M., et al. (2002) CXCR4/CXCL12 expression and signalling in kidney cancer. *Br J Cancer.*, **86**, 1250–6.

95. Haviv Y. S., van Houdt W. J., Lu B., et al. (2004) Transcriptional targeting in renal cancer cell lines via the human CXCR4 promoter. *Mol Cancer Ther*. **3**, 687–91.
96. Pan J., Mestas J., Burdick M. D., et al. (2006) Stromal derived factor-1 (SDF-1/ CXCL12) and CXCR4 in renal cell carcinoma metastasis. *Mol Cancer*. **5**, 56.
97. Jones J., Marian D., Weich E., et al. (2007) CXCR4 chemokine receptor engagement modifies integrin dependent adhesion of renal carcinoma cells. *Exp Cell Res.*, **313**, 4051–65.
98. Sehgal A., Keener C., Boynton A. L., et al. (1998) CXCR-4, a chemokine receptor, is overexpressed in and required for proliferationof glioblastoma tumor cells. *J Surg Oncol.*, **69**, 99–104.
99. Sehgal A., Ricks S., Boynton A. L., et al. (1998) Molecular characterization of CXCR-4: A potential brain tumor-associated gene. *J Surg Oncol.*, **69**, 239–48.
100. Rempel S. A., Dudas S., Ge S., and Gutiérrez J. A. (2000) Identification and localization of the cytokine SDF1 and its receptor, CXC chemokine receptor 4, to regions of necrosis and angiogenesis in human glioblastoma. *Clin Cancer Res.* **6**, 102–11.
101. Rubin J. B., Kung A. L., Klein R. S., et al. (2003) A small-molecule antagonist of CXCR4 inhibits intracranial growth of primary brain tumors. *Proc Natl Acad Sci U S A*. **100**, 13513–8.
102. Salmaggi A., Gelati M., Pollo B., et al. (2004) CXCL12 in malignant glial tumors: a possible role in angiogenesis and cross-talk between endothelial and tumoral cells. *J Neurooncol.* **67**, 305–17.
103. Schüller U., Koch A., Hartmann W., et al. (2005) Subtype-specific expression and genetic alterations of the chemokinereceptor gene CXCR4 in medulloblastomas. *Int J Cancer.*, **117**, s82–9.
104. Ping Y. F., Yao X. H., Chen J. H., et al. (2007) The anti-cancer compound Nordy inhibits CXCR4-mediated production of IL-8 and VEGF by malignant human glioma cells. *J Neurooncol.*, **84**, 21–9.
105. Bian X. W., Yang S. X., Chen J. H., et al. (2007) Preferential expression of chemokine receptor CXCR4 by highly malignant human gliomas and its association with poor patient survival. *Neurosurgery*, **61**, 570–8.
106. Borrello M. G., Alberti L., Fischer A., et al. (2005) Induction of a proinflammatory program in normal human thyrocytes by the RET/PTC1 oncogene. *Proc Natl Acad Sci U S A*. **102**, 14825–30.
107. De Falco V., Guarino V., Avilla E., et al. (2007) Biological role and potential therapeutic targeting of the chemokine receptor CXCR4 in undifferentiated thyroid cancer. *Cancer Res.*, **67**, 11821–9.
108. Koshiba T., Hosotani R., Miyamoto Y., et al. (2000) Expression of stromal cell-derived factor 1 and CXCR4 ligand receptor system in pancreatic cancer: A possible role for tumor progression. *Clin Cancer Res.*, **6**, 3530–5.
109. Mori T., Doi R., Koizumi M., et al. (2004) CXCR4 antagonist inhibits stromal cell-derived factor 1-induced migration and invasion of human pancreatic cancer. *Mol Cancer Ther.*, **3**, 29–37.
110. Sato N., Fukushima N., Maitra A., et al. (2004) Gene expression profiling identifies genes associated with invasive intraductal papillary mucinous neoplasms of the pancreas. *Am J Pathol*. **164**, 903–14.
111. Marchesi F., Monti P., Leone B. E., et al. (2004) Increased survival, proliferation, and migration in metastatic human pancreatic tumor cells expressing functional CXCR4. *Cancer Res.*, **64**, 8420–7.
112. Wehler T., Wolfert F., Schimanski C. C., et al. (2006) Strong expression of chemokine receptor CXCR4 by pancreatic cancer correlates with advanced disease. *Oncol Rep.*, **16**, 1159–64.
113. Billadeau D. D., Chatterjee S., Bramati P., et al. (2006) Characterization of the CXCR4 signaling in pancreatic cancer cells. *Int J Gastrointest Cancer.*, **37**, 110–9.

114. Kaifi J. T., Yekebas E. F., Schurr P., et al. (2005) Tumor-cell homing to lymph nodes and bone marrow and CXCR4 expression in esophageal cancer. *J Natl Cancer Inst* **97**, 1840–7.

115. Koishi K., Yoshikawa R., Tsujimura T., et al.. (2006) Persistent CXCR4 expression after preoperative chemoradiotherapy predicts early recurrence and poor prognosis in esophageal cancer. *World J Gastroenterol.*, **12**, 7585–90.

116. Gockel I., Schimanski C. C., Heinrich C., et al. (2006) Expression of chemokine receptor CXCR4 in esophageal squamous cell and adenocarcinoma. *BMC Cancer.*, **6**, 290.

117. Kodama J., Hasengaowa, Kusumoto T., et al. (2007) Association of CXCR4 and CCR7 chemokine receptor expression and lymph node metastasis in human cervical cancer. *Ann Oncol.*, **18**, 70–6.

118. Zhang J. P., Lu W. G., Ye F., et al. (2007) Study on CXCR4/SDF-1alpha axis in lymph node metastasis of cervical squamous cell carcinoma. *Int J Gynecol Cancer.*, **17**, 478–83.

119. Yang Y. C., Lee Z. Y., Wu C. C., et al. (2007) CXCR4 expression is associated with pelvic lymph node metastasis in cervical adenocarcinoma. *Int J Gynecol Cancer.*, **17**, 676–86.

120. Almofti A., Uchida D., Begum N. M., et al. (2004) The clinicopathological significance of the expression of CXCR4 protein in oral squamous cell carcinoma. *Int J Oncol.*, **25**, 65–71.

121. Uchida D., Begum N. M., Tomizuka Y., et al. (2004) Acquisition of lymph node, but not distant metastatic potentials, by the overexpression of CXCR4 in human oral squamous cell carcinoma. *Lab Invest.* b, 1538–46.

122. Ishikawa T., Nakashiro K., Hara S., et al. (2006) CXCR4 expression is associated with lymph-node metastasis of oral squamous cell carcinoma. *Int J Oncol.* **28**, 61–6.

123. Onoue T., Uchida D., Begum N. M., et al.(2006) Epithelial-mesenchymal transition induced by the stromal cell-derived factor-1/CXCR4 system in oral squamous cell carcinoma cells. *Int J Oncol.*, **29**, 1133–8.

124. Li H., Alizadeh H., and Niederkorn J. Y. (2008) Differential expression of chemokine receptors on uveal melanoma cells and their metastases. *Invest Ophthalmol Vis Sci.*, **49**, 636–43.

125. Di Cesare S., Marshall J. C., Fernandes B. F., et al. (2007) In vitro characterization and inhibition of the CXCR4/CXCL12 chemokine axis in human uveal melanoma cell lines. *Cancer Cell Int.*, **7**, 17.

126. Tucci M. G., Lucarini G., Brancorsini D., et al. (2007) Involvement of E-cadherin, beta-catenin, Cdc42 and CXCR4 in the progression and prognosis of cutaneous melanoma. *Br J Dermatol.* **157**, 1212–6.

127. Schutyser E., Su Y., Yu Y., et al. (2007) Hypoxia enhances CXCR4 expression in human microvascular endothelial cells and human melanoma cells. *Eur Cytokine Netw.* **18**, 59–70.

128. Robledo M. M., Bartolome R. A., Longo N., et al. (2001) Expression of functional chemokine receptors CXCR3 and CXCR4 on human melanoma cells. *J Biol Chem.* **276**, 45098–105.

129. Payne A. S. and Cornelius L. A. (2002) The role of chemokines in melanoma tumor growth and metastasis. *J Invest Dermatol.*, **118**, 915–22.

130. Murakami T., Maki W., Cardones A. R., et al. (2002) Expression of CXC chemokine receptor-4 enhances the pulmonary metastatic potential of murine B16 melanoma cells. *Cancer Res.*, **62**, 7328–34.

131. Scala S., Ottaiano A., Ascierto P. A., et al. (2005) Expression of CXCR4 predicts poor prognosis in patients with malignant melanoma. *Clin Cancer Res.* **11**, 1835–41.

132. Longo-Imedio M. I., Longo N., Treviño I., et al.(2005) Clinical significance of CXCR3 and CXCR4 expression in primary melanoma. *Int J Cancer.*, **117**, 861–5.

133. Möhle R., Bautz F., Rafii S., et al. (1998) The chemokine receptor CXCR-4 is expressed on CD34+ hematopoietic progenitors and leukemic cells and mediates transendothelial migration induced by stromal cell-derived factor-1. Bilood, **91**, 4523–30.

134. Burger J. A., Burger M., and Kipps T. J. (1999) Chronic lymphocytic leukemia B cells express functional CXCR4 chemokine receptors that mediate spontaneous migration beneath bone marrow stromal cells. *Blood*, **94**, 3658–67.

135. Sipkins D. A., Wei X., Wu J. W., et al. (2005) In vivo imaging of specialized bone marrow endothelial microdomains for tumour engraftment. *Nature*, 435, 969–73.

136. Monaco G., Belmont J. W., Konopleva M., et al. (2004) Correlation between CXCR4 and homing or engraftment of acute myelogenous leukemia. *Cancer Res.* **64**, 6832.

137. Dommange F., Cartron G., Espanel C., et al. (2006) CXCL12 polymorphism and malignant cell dissemination/tissue infiltration in acute myeloid leukemia. *FASEB J.* **20**, 1913–5.

138. Kalinkovich A., Tavor S., Avigdor A., et al. (2006) Functional CXCR4-expressing microparticles and SDF-1 correlate with circulating acute myelogenous leukemia cells. *Cancer* Ries. **66**, 11013–20.

139. Konoplev S., Rassidakis G. Z., Estey E., et al. (2007) Overexpression of CXCR4 predicts adverse overall and event-free survival in patients with unmutated FLT3 acute myeloid leukemia with normal karyotype. *Cancer*, **109**, 1152–6.

140. Zeelenberg I. S., Ruuls-Van Stalle L., and Roos E. (2001) Retention of CXCR4 in the endoplasmic reticulum blocks dissemination of a T cell hybridoma. *JClin Invest.*, **108**, 269–77.

HIF-1 Regulation of Chemokine Receptor Expression

Elizabeth W. Newcomb and David Zagzag

Abstract The chemokine-chemokine receptor system is a highly conserved family of small molecules that bind to a given receptor(s) to regulate the mobilization and trafficking of cells. Hypoxia within the tumor microenvironment plays a role in the upregulation of several chemokine receptors on tumor cells and secretion of different chemokines promoting tumor cell invasion and metastatic spread. Preliminary data from animal models show promising antitumor efficacy with the use of small molecule chemokine receptor antagonists to prevent tumor growth and metastasis. Future studies are needed to evaluate chemokine receptor antagonists alone and in combination with other standard radiation and chemotherapy regimens to control not only local tumor growth but also metastatic potential.

Introduction

New treatment options for human cancers as well as a better understanding of their physiological and molecular nature are essential to improving the clinical outcome of patients. Cytokines have, to a great extent, the power to mobilize and activate intracellular signaling pathways that are critical for tumor progression. One regulator of chemokine receptor expression is hypoxia-inducible factor-1 (HIF-1), a heterodimeric transcription factor regulating O_2 concentration in tissues and whose activation is dependent on the relative abundance of cellular O_2 levels. HIF-1 is responsible for upregulating many genes containing hypoxic response elements (HREs) and plays a major role in chemokine-chemokine receptor systems. In this chapter we will summarize the modulating effect of HIF-1 on chemokine receptor expression, including CXCR1, CXCR2,

E.W. Newcomb (✉)
Department of Pathology, New York University Cancer Institute, New York University School of Medicine, New York, NY 10016, USA
e-mail: newcoe01@med.nyu.edu

A.M. Fulton (ed.), *Chemokine Receptors in Cancer*, Cancer Drug Discovery and Development, DOI 10.1007/978-1-60327-267-4_3,

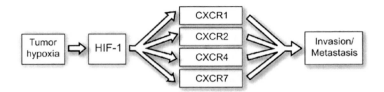

Fig. 1 The schema indicates how hypoxia may play a role in the upregulation of chemokine receptors in tumors and its role in promoting tumor cell invasion and metastases. Tumor hypoxia upregulates HIF-1 that in turn sets in motion an adaptive response regulated by a large number of molecules including the chemokine receptors CXCR1, CXCR2, CXCR4, and CXCR7. Hypoxia also upregulates expression of the pro-angiogenic factors VEGF and CXCL8. Exposure of endothelial cells to VEGF can induce expression of the chemokines CXCL1, CXCL8, and CXCL12. CXCL1 ligand signals only through CXCR2, CXCL8 signals through both CXCR1 and CXCR2, and CXCL12 signals through both CXCR4 and CXCR7. Therefore, turning on expression and secretion of different chemokines from blood vessels would form chemokine gradients attracting chemokine receptor-positive hypoxic tumor cells to migrate toward the chemokine-positive blood vessels or promote trafficking to other organs overexpressing similar chemokines

CXCR4, and CXCR7 (Fig. 1). Novel potential therapeutic targeting of chemokine receptors to inhibit local tumor growth and decrease the potential for metastasis will be discussed.

Hypoxia-Inducible Factor-1

Hypoxia-inducible factor-1 (HIF-1) is a heterodimeric basic-helix-loop-helix-PAS transcription factor that regulates O_2 concentrations in tissues [29, 76, 78, 93]. HIF-1 consists of two subunits, HIF-1α and HIF-1β (also called aryl hydrocarbon nuclear translocator, ARNT). The activation of HIF-1 transcriptional activity is dependent on the relative abundance of cellular levels of O_2 and stabilization of the HIF-1α subunit [34, 36, 78]. The HIF-1β subunit is constitutively expressed compared with the HIF-1α subunit, whose abundance is decreased in normoxic conditions but markedly increased during hypoxic conditions. The levels of the HIF-1α subunit are controlled through degradation by the proteasome [35, 38, 72, 78]. Binding of the von Hippel-Lindau tumor-suppressor protein (VHL) to the HIF-1α subunit recruits the protein Elongin C and the E3 ubiquitin-protein ligase complex that uibiquinates HIF-1α targeting it for proteasomal degradation. The binding of VHL is controlled by hydroxylation of prolyl residues by the prolyl hydroxylase domain protein 2 (PHD2), an activity which is reduced under hypoxic conditions [78]. Thus, degradation of HIF-1α by the proteasome is inhibited and HIF-1α protein accumulates allowing dimerization with the HIF-1β subunit and increased HIF-1 transcriptional activity. HIF-1 upregulates the expression of many genes that contain HREs, such as vascular endothelial growth factor (VEGF), a highly potent cytokine known to promote angiogenesis [17, 25], and the chemokine receptor CXCR4 and its ligand stromal cell-derived factor-1α (SDF-1α, CXCL12) [83, 74, 105].

The Chemokine-Chemokine Receptor System

The chemokine-chemokine receptor system is a highly conserved family of small molecules that bind to a given receptor(s) to regulate the mobilization and trafficking of cells within an organism. Currently, 53 human chemokines and 23 chemokine receptors have been identified ([113]; http://cytokine. medic.kumamoto-u.ac.jp/). The nomenclature for the genes has been standardized and the genes have been grouped based on their protein structures. The chemokines consist mainly of two major groups according to the positions of the N-terminal cysteine residues: CC, are adjacent whereas CXC has one amino acid in between. However, there are two exceptions. One chemokine, XCL1 (lymphotactin), lacks the typical cysteines at position one and three, while the other chemokine, CX3C (fractalkine), contains three amino acids between the cysteines. The standardized names of each gene incorporate an "L" referring to the chemokine ligands or an "R" referring to the chemokine receptors. For example, the ligand CXCL12 for SDF-1 binds to its cognate receptor CXCR4. The chemokine receptors contain seven-transmembrane domains similar to G-protein-coupled cell surface receptors. The two major groups of chemokine receptors are designated CXCR1-7 and CCR1-16. One chemokine may bind to several receptors and similarly one chemokine receptor may induce signaling for several chemokines. Another level of complexity within the chemokine-chemokine-receptor system comes from the fact that many cell types express more than one chemokine receptor.

HIF-1 Dependent and Independent Pathways
for VEGF-Induced Angiogenesis

As mentioned previously, HIF-1 transcriptional activity upregulates the expression of many genes to allow adaptation of cells to different microenvironments. One gene whose expression is regulated by HIF-1 is the cytokine VEGF. Stimulation of vascular endothelial cells by VEGF induces the formation of new blood vessels from pre-exising host blood vessels, a process called neovascularization. Although the expression of HIF-1 and VEGF is commonly associated with angiogenesis in the development and progression of tumors [31, 76, 105], there are a number of other processes that also involve angiogenesis. These include neovascularization associated with the development of organs, tissue repair after ischemia, wound healing, and inflammation [27, 41, 53, 62, 65, 82, 89].

The cytokine VEGF can also be induced by several HIF-1 independent pathways [53]. The angiogenic factor interleukin 8 (IL-8, CXCL8) has been associated with induction of VEGF expression in hypoxic tumors lacking HIF-1. The transcription factor nuclear factor-κB (NF-κB) can regulate VEGF directly as well as indirectly in response to hypoxic conditions. NF-κB can also induce HIF-1 under certain conditions in response to reactive oxygen species (ROS) and stimulation by interleukin-1β (IL-1β) [9, 37]. Importantly, NF-κB can induce expression of the angiogenic factor CXCL8 through a HIF-1-independent pathway [52]. Both VEGF and CXCL8, whether induced by HIF-1 dependent or independent pathways, regulate the expression of several chemokine receptors.

Hypoxia and Upregulation of Chemokine Receptors CXCR1 and CXCR2 Expression

The chemokine receptors CXCR1 and CXCR2 bind to the ligand CXCL8 [113]. The chemokine CXCL8 plays a role in leukocyte trafficking, inflammation, and angiogenesis [12]. Several studies have shown regulation of CXCR1 and CXCR2 in normal vascular endothelial cells and cardiomyocytes by hypoxia [28, 54]. However, CXCL8 and expression of its receptors CXCR1 and CXCR2 are now increasingly associated with the development and progression of many human tumors [99]. In glioblastoma tumor specimens, CXCL8 showed increased expression in hypoxic regions of the tumor [22]. Expression of the CXCR1 and CXCR2 receptors for CXCL8 occurs on human microvascular endothelial cells (HMECs). CXCL8 induces migration of HMECs that would play a critical role in mediating angiogenic activity, similar to that described below for the CXCL12 ligand and its receptor CXCR4.

Recently the upregulation of the CXCR1 and CXCR2 receptors in human prostate PC3 cancer cells by hypoxia was reported [50]. Both HIF-1 and NF-κB were shown to play a role in CXCR1 and CXCR2 receptor expression since inhibition of either HIF-1 or NF-κB through siRNA knockdown technology inhibited the expression of both chemokine receptors. CXCL8 was also induced by hypoxia concurrently with the chemokine receptors that may serve as an autocrine/paracrine signaling pathway for hypoxic tumor cells. Due to the role of CXCL8 in regulating angiogenesis, the coordinated upregulation of CXCL8 with its receptors may promote prostate tumor growth and progression as all three proteins have been detected in prostate cancer specimens [56].

Tumor invasion in head and neck tumors has been associated with secretion of chemokines CXCL1 and CXCL8 by the endothelial cells promoting invasion of CXCR2 receptor positive tumor cells [95]. Endothelial cells exposed to VEGF-induced expression of the chemokines CXCL1 and CXCL8. Since CXCL8 signals through both CXCR1 and CXCR2 receptors, whereas CXCL1 signals only through CXCR2, antibodies directed against CXCR2 inhibited the invasion of the tumor cells. The prosurvival factor Bcl-2 induces both CXCL1 and CXCL8 expression through NF-κB. VEGF also induced

Bcl-2 and endothelial cells engineered to overexpress Bcl-2 show overexpression of CXCL1 and CXCL8. The endothelial cells in patients with head and neck squamous cell carcinoma (HNSCC) show markedly high expression of Bcl-2 compared with normal endothelial cells. Through both in vitro and in vivo studies, overexpression of Bcl-2 by endothelial cells was directly correlated with their production of CXCL1 and CXCL8 and signaling through CXCR2 on the tumor cells.

Some of the known CXC chemokines have a conserved motif in the N-terminus, Glu-Leu-Arg (ELR +) and these chemokines are pro-angiogenic compared with ELR- chemokines which are anti-angiogenic [86]. Among the ELR + chemokines are CXCL8, granulocyte chemotactic protein-2 (GCP-2, CXCL6), and epithelial neutrophil-activating protein-78 (ENA-78). All the ELR + chemokines, except CXCL8 and CXCL6 (GCP-2) that bind to the CXCR1 receptor, signal through the CXCR2 receptor [86]. Small cell lung cancers (SCLCs) express both CXCR1 and CXCR2 receptors [112]. A recent study demonstrated that hypoxia and IL-1β can significantly upregulate the expression of CXCL6 [112]. NF-κB was identified as the major transcription factor mediating CXCL6 expression, but IL-2β also upregulated CXCL6. Hypoxia increased secretion of CXCL6 in SCLC cells and this was mediated by HIF-1 due to the presence of a potential HRE in the promoter region of CXCL6.

In summary, the chemokines CXCL1, CXCL6, and CXCL8 that bind to CXCR1 and CXCR2 receptors and the receptors themselves can be regulated by hypoxia through both HIF-1-dependent and -independent pathways.

Hypoxia and Upregulation of Chemokine Receptor CXCR7 Expression

Recently an alternate receptor, CXCR7, for the chemokine CXCL12 was identified and characterized [15]. It was found expressed on many tumor cell lines, on activated endothelial cells, and restricted in its expression on normal cells to fetal liver cells. It differs from many other chemokine receptors, particularly CXCR4, which also binds to the same ligand (CXCL12), where binding of ligand activates CXCR7 without inducing cell migration [15]. Expression of CXCR7 appears to be associated with increasing cell survival and adhesion of CXCR7-positive tumor cells to activated CXCR7-positive endothelial cells [15]. Since many tumor cell types overexpress CXCR7, the CXCR7 antagonist CCX754 was evaluated for its efficacy to inhibit the growth of tumors in both immunnodeficient and immunocompetent animal models [15]. Thus, the CXCR7 receptor, similar to CXCR4, the other CXCL12-binding receptor CXCR4, can serve as a therapeutic target for human cancers.

CXCR7 is expressed in a wide variety of human cancer cell lines, including breast, cervical, lymphoma, glioma, and lung [15]. Studies of human malignancies show that CXCR7 is expressed in breast, lung, prostate, rhabdomyosarcoma, cervical squamous cell carcinoma, and renal cell carcinoma [53, 94]. In prostate cancer, CXCR7 expression is correlated with increasing tumor grade and promotes invasion in animal models [94]. Inflammatory cytokines TNF-α and IL-1β regulate the expression of CXCR7 on endothelial cells which may enhance the adhesion of tumor cells to the tumor vasculature [15, 44]. Prostate cells engineered to overexpress CXCR7 secreted more CXCL8 and VEGF. Exposure of CXCR7-overexpressing cells to CXCL12 also increased secretion of IL-8 and VEGF. Conditioned medium from CXCR7-overexpresssing cells increased tubule formation in endothelial cell cultures showing that the pro-angiogenic factors played a role in angiogenesis [94]. Both knockdown studies of CXCR7 and use of specific CXCR7 antagonists have shown inhibition of tumor growth in vivo in several animal models [15, 53, 94]. Although definitive studies have yet to evaluate whether HIF-1 plays a role in regulating the expression of CXCR7, the fact that CXCR7-overexpressing cells produce two pro-angiogenic chemokines, CXCL8 and VEGF, suggest that its expression may be regulated by both HIF-1-dependent and - independent pathways, possibly involving NF-κB signaling as noted above.

Hypoxia and Upregulation of Chemokine Receptor CXCR4 Expression in Glioma

The chemokine-chemokine receptor system regulated by HIF-1 and the one most studied in relation to organogenesis, tissue repair, tumorigenesis, and metastasis is CXCL12 ligand and its receptor CXCR4 [5, 14, 16, 19, 43, 44, 45, 47, 62, 65, 70, 114, 115]. The expression of CXCR4 has been observed as a common finding in more than 29 human cancers (Table 1) and correlated with increasing malignancy and aggressive growth. Recent evidence has established that CXCR4 expression regulates metastatic potential in breast and renal cell cancers by upregulating genes such as urokinase-type plasminogen activator receptor and metalloproteinases, respectively [79, 87]. Since the human cancers with CXCR4 and CXCL12 expression have hypoxic tumor microenvironments similar to glioma, we will focus on how CXCR4 expression is regulated by HIF-1 in glioma and is associated with invasion [106, 107].

Unlike other cancers where tumor cells from the primary location spread to metastatic sites, gliomas invade locally throughout the brain tissue adjacent to the tumor. We have proposed that the CXCL12/CXCR4 axis was important in the directional invasion of glioma cells into the neighboring parenchyma.

The mechanisms of the hypoxia-mediated invasion in gliomas have been partially elucidated [11, 64, 77, 105]. However, it is known that hypoxia stimulates tumor cell migration in vitro and tumor cell invasion and metastasis in vivo [10, 77, 84]. HIF-1α is commonly observed at the invading margins of human and murine cancers [104, 111]. For example, GFP labeling of GL261 glioma cells identified most HIF-1α-expressing cells as those invading into the surrounding brain [104]. HIF-1 upregulates a variety of genes whose products

Table 1 Tumors that express CXCR4 and relation to prognosis and metastatic disease

Tumor type	*References
Bladder cancer	[68]
Breast cancer	*[5], *[70, 80, 98]
Cervical cancer	[40, 101, 108]
Colon cancer	*[26, 59, 70]
Esophageal	*[70]
Gastric cancer	*[70, 102]
Glioblastoma	*[4, 5, 8, 106, 107]
Head and neck	[55]
Hematopoietic	
B-CLL	*[5], *[14]
Multiple myeloma	[2, 90]
B-cell lymphomas	[63]
Acute leukemias	*[5], *[14]
AML	*[5], *[14]
Hepatocellular	[73]
Kidney cancer	*[5]
Lung cancer	
NSCLC	*[70, 88]
SCLC	*[5]
Nasopharyngeal	*[60, 70]
Neuroblastoma	*[5, 71]
Oral squamous carcinoma	*[5, 21, 92]
Ovarian cancer	*[5]
Osteosarcoma	*[57, 70]
Pancreatic cancer	*[5, 96]
Prostate cancer	*[1, 5]
Renal cell carcinoma	[61, 83, 87]
Rhabdomyosarcoma	[85]
Skin cancer	
Melanoma	*[5], *[70, 75, 91]
Non-melanoma	[7]
Thyroid carcinoma	[18]

*References include review articles citing older literature
with updated references for a given tumor type.

play a well-established role in glioma invasion [11, 42, 64, 104, 106]. These
include CXCR4, CXCL12, VEGF, MMP-2, and MMP-9 [23, 42]. Previous
studies by our group and others suggest that hypoxia stimulates glioma cell
migration in vitro and invasion in orthotopic glioma models and human
gliomas [11, 64, 104, 106].

Abundant experimental evidence suggests that the CXCR4/CXCL12 pathway
is a crucial component of invasion in gliomas. Glioma cell lines overexpress
CXCR4 and CXCL12. CXCL12 has been shown to exert proliferative, anti-
apoptotic, and chemotactic effects on glioma cell lines in vitro. Primary human
gliomas expressed CXCR4 and CXCL12 in glioma cells [6, 58, 67, 69, 97, 106, 110].

We and others have shown that hypoxia and HIF-1α upregulate CXCR4 mRNA and protein in glioma cells and stressed the role of CXCR4 in glioma cell invasion [3, 24, 33, 97, 105, 109]. For example, CXCR4-expressing human and rodent glioma cells demonstrate enhanced invasive capacity as compared to noninvasive tumor cells in vitro and in vivo [24]. We have previously shown that when exposed to hypoxia, glioma cells in which HIF-1α expression was inhibited by RNA interference failed to show HIF-1α and CXCR4 upregulation under hypoxic conditions while CXCR4 inhibition prevented migration [106].

Moreover, the capacity of CXCR4 to mobilize tumor cells has been linked to increased production of MMPs [81]. MMPs are known to be overexpressed in gliomas, and their production has been shown to promote glioma cell invasiveness [46]. These studies indicate that the hypoxia and HIF-1-induction of CXCR4, the engagement of the CXCR4 receptor by CXCL12, and CXCR4 signaling may mediate glioma invasion, at least in part, directly through upregulation of MMP production [4, 24, 33, 106, 109].

In summary, recent data support the hypothesis that migration of glioma cells at the edge of gliomas is not random but may relate to the differential expression of CXCL12 and CXCR4 at the invading edge of gliomas to drive invasion into the brain parenchyma [107]. Hypoxia induces local migration by upregulating CXCR4 in glioma cells, and by inducing VEGF secretion which in turn leads to upregulation of CXCL12 by blood vessels. Therefore, turning on CXCL12 expression and its secretion from blood vessels would form a CXCL12 gradient attracting CXCR4-positive glioma cells from the tumor core to migrate toward the CXCL12-positive blood vessels in the brain adjacent to the tumor. Thus, hypoxia-induced expression of functional CXCR4 receptors by glioma cells together with VEGF-induced upregulation of CXCL12 may represent one molecular basis for brain tumor dispersal. Inhibition of CXCR4/CXCL12 interactions by small molecule antagonists, such as AMD3100, or shRNA knockdown technology, could potentially control the invasive behavior of glioma cells, decreasing invasion of cells into the brain parenchyma and improving the prognosis of patients with gliomas.

Potential Therapeutic Targeting of Chemokine Receptors to Inhibit Tumor Growth

The tumor microenvironment plays a critical role in tumor progression and metastasis. Both chemokine receptors CXCR4 and CXCR7 are overexpressed in a wide number of human malignancies and both bind the same ligand CXCL12 that serves as a potent chemoattractant for tumor cells promoting invasion and/or metastasis. Although tumor hypoxia regulates expression of HIF-1 to induce secretion of the chemokine VEGF and promote angiogenesis, production of inflammatory cytokines by macrophages or stimuli such as ROS, radiation or chemotherapy treatments can induce VEGF by HIF-1-independent means.

As noted above, CXCR4 expression is regulated by hypoxia in many human tumors, and thus would serve as a potential therapeutic target for inhibiting tumor growth.

Several studies using animal models have now validated that small molecule antagonists of CXCR4 or CXCR7 [15, 20, 39, 66, 69, 100, 103], or knock down of CXCR4 or CXCR7 expression with siRNA technology [30, 49, 51, 94] can inhibit tumor growth.

The bicyclam antagonist of CXCR4 activation AMD3100 and a newer generation competitive antagonist AMD4365, with higher affinity for CXCR4 and greater solubility in water, have been used in animal models of glioma and medulloblastoma brain tumors [69, 100]. Delivery of AMD3100 to animals with established orthotopic intracranial tumors by daily subcutaneous injection or by osmotic pumps for 3–5 weeks inhibited tumor growth [69, 100]. Inhibition of growth was associated with increased apoptosis and decreased activation of Erk 1/2 and phosphatidylinositol3-kinase (PI3K) signaling pathway. The results of this study showed that both AMD3100 and AMD4365 could pass the blood-brain barrier to effectively inhibit tumor growth. Other studies in similar glioma tumor models tested the efficacy of combining AMD3100 with subtherapeutic doses of the alkylating agent BCNU [66]. Combination treatment resulted in synergistic inhibition of tumor growth, indicating that this approach may be clinically relevant for brain tumor patients. Thyroid cancer also overexpresses CXCR4 [20]. Animal models of human anaplastic thyroid xenografts treated with AMD3100 by daily intraperitoneal injection for 3–4 weeks showed significant antitumor efficacy that was correlated with increased cell death rather than a decrease in blood vessels and an anti-angiogenic effect.

The peptide CXCR4 antagonist TN14003 has demonstrated antitumor efficacy in two animal models of metastatic breast and head and neck cancer [48, 103]. Animals were treated with the CXCR4 peptide by intraperitoneal injection for 35 days. Tumors at the primary subcutaneous site of injection as well as the number of lung metastasis were inhibited. In the head and neck animal model, antitumor activity was correlated with anti-angiogenic activity of the anti-CXCR4 treatment.

Using two murine models of metastatic osteosarcoma and melanoma the small peptide CXCR4 antagonist CTCE-9908, a 17-amino acid analog of CXCL12, inhibited lung metastasis after tail vein injection of the tumor cells [39]. Studies performed in vitro demonstrated that exposure of tumor cells to CTCE-9908 decreased adhesion, migration, invasion, and proliferation. Taken together, these properties were associated with the inhibition of tumor growth observed in vivo. Similar to AMD3100, CTCE-9908 is currently being tested in clinical trials [39].

In summary, small molecule peptide antagonists of CXCR4 and CXCR7 have shown promising antitumor efficacy in several animal models of human cancer with a good toxicity profile. Currently, an appropriate clinical approach for antagonizing CXCR4 and CXCR7 remains unknown. AMD3100 is currently used for mobilizing bone marrow stem cells in patients with multiple myeloma and non-Hodgkin's lymphoma prior to autologous bone marrow transplantation [13, 23]. Toxicity studies of AMD3100 show prolonged treatment over 10 days produced mild toxicity related to its effects on bone marrow function [32]. Future studies are required to continue to evaluate antagonists directed against CXCR4 and CXCR7, their use as monotherapies or in combination with standard radiation, and chemotherapy regimens to control not only local tumor growth but also to decrease metastatic potential.

References

1. Akashi T, Koizumi K, Tsuneyama K, et al. (2008) Chemokine receptor CXCR4 expression and prognosis in patients with metastatic prostate cancer. Cancer Sci 99:539–542
2. Alsayed Y, Ngo H, Runnels J, et al. (2007) Mechanisms of regulation of CXCR4/SDF-1 (CXCL12)-dependent migration and homing in multiple myeloma. Blood 7:2708–2717
3. Bajetto A, Barbero S, Bonavia R, et al. (2001) Stromal cell-derived factor- 1alpha induces astrocyte proliferation through the activation of extracellular signal-regulated kinases ½ pathway.J Neurochem 77:1226–1236
4. Bajetto A, Barbieri F, Dorcaratto A, et al. (2006) Expression of CXC chemokine receptors 1-5 and their ligands in human glioma tissues: Role of CXCR4 and SDF1 in glioma cell proliferation and migration. Neurochem Int 49:423–432
5. Balkwill F (2004) The significance of cancer cell expression of the chemokine receptor CXCR4. Sem Cancer Biol 14:171–179
6. Barbero S, Bonavia R, Bajetto A, et al. (2003) Stromal cell-derived factor 1a stimulates human glioblastoma cell growth through the activation of both extracellular signal-regulated kinases ½ and Akt. Cancer Res 63:1969–1974
7. Basile J, Thiers B, Maize J, et al. (2008) Chemokine receptor expression in non-melanoma skin cancer. J Cutan Pathol DOI:10.1111/j.1600-0560.2007.00879.x
8. Bian X, Yang S, Chen J, et al. (2007) Preferential expression of chemokine receptor CXCR4 by highly malignant human gliomas and its association with poor patient survival. Neurosurgery 61:570–579
9. Bonello S, Zähringer C, BelAiba RS, et al. (2007) Reactive oxygen species activate the HIF-1alpha promoter via a functional NFkappaB site. Arterioscler Thromb Vasc Biol 27:755–761
10. Bottaro DP and Liotta LA (2003) Cancer: Out of air is not out of action. Nature 423:593–595
11. Brat DJ, Castellano-Sanchez AA, Hunter SB, et al. (2004) Pseudopalisades in glioblastoma are hypoxic, express extracellular matrix proteases, and are formed by an actively migrating cell population. Cancer Res 64:920–927
12. Brat DJ, Bellail AC, Van Meir EG (2005) The role of interleukin-8 and its receptors in gliomagenesis and tumoral angiogenesis. Neuro-Oncol 7:122–133
13. Broxmeyer HE, Orschell CM, Clapp DW, et al. (2005) Rapid mobilization of murine and human hematopoietic stem and progenitor cells with AMD3100, a CXCR4 antagonist. J Exp Med 201:1307–1318
14. Burger JA and Kipps TJ (2005) CXCR4: A key receptor in the crosstalk between tumor cells and their microenvironment. Blood 107:1761–1767
15. Burns JM, Summers BC, Wang Y, et al. (2006) A novel chemokine receptor for SDF-1 and I-TAC involved in cell survival, cell adhesion, and tumor development. J Exp Med 203:2201–2213

16. Busillo JM and Benovic JL (2007) Regulation of CXCR4 signaling. Biochim Biophys Acta Biomembranes 1768:952–963
17. Carmeliet P, Dor Y, Herbert JM, et al. (1998) Role of HIF-1alpha in hypoxia-mediated apoptosis, cell proliferation and tumour angiogenesis. Nature 394:485–490
18. Castellone M, Guarino V, De Falco V, et al. (2004) Functional expression of the CXCR4 chemokine receptor is induced by RET/PTC oncogenes and is a common event in human papillary thyroid carcinomas. Oncogene 23:5958–5967
19. Ceradini DJ, Kulkarni AR, Callaghan MJ, et al. (2004) Progenitor cell trafficking is regulated by hypoxic gradients through HIF-1 induction of SDF-1. Nat Med 10: 858–864
20. De Falco V, Guarino V, Avilla E, et al. (2007) Biological role and potential therapeutic targeting of the chemokine receptor CXCR4 in undifferentiated thyroid cancer. Cancer Res 67:11821–11829
21. Delilbasi C, Okura M, Iidam S, et al. (2004) Investigation of CXCR4 in squamous cell carcinoma of the tongue. Oral Oncology 40:154–157
22. Desbaillets I, Diserens AC, de Tribolet N, et al. (1997) Upregulation of interleukin 8 by oxygen-deprived cells in glioblastoma suggests a role in leukocyte activation, chemotaxis, and angiogenesis. J Exp Med 186:1201–1212
23. Devine SM, Flomenberg N, Vesole DH, et al. (2004) Rapid mobilization of CD34 + cells following administration of the CXCR4 antagonist AMD3100 to patients with multiple myeloma and non-Hodgkin's lymphoma. J Clin Oncol 22:1095–1020
24. Ehtesham M, Winston JA, Kabos P, et al. (2006) CXCR4 expression mediates glioma cell invasiveness. Oncogene 25:2801–2806
25. Forsythe JA, Jiang BH, Iyer NV, et al. (1996) Activation of vascular endothelial growth factor gene transcription by hypoxia-inducible factor 1. Mol Cell Biol 16:4604–4613
26. Fukunaga S, Maeda K, Noda E, et al. (2006) Association between expression of vascular endothelial growth factor C, chemokine receptor CXCR4 and lymph node metastasis in colorectal cancer. Oncology 71:204–211
27. Galiano RD, Tepper OM, Pelo CR, et al. (2004) Topical vascular endothelial growth factor accelerates diabetic wound healing through increased angiogenesis and by mobilizing and recruiting bone marrow-derived cells. Am J Pathol 164:1935–1947
28. Grutkoski PS, Graeber CT, D'Amico R, et al. (1999) Regulation of IL-8RA (CXCR1) expression in polymorphonucler leukocytes by hypoxia/reoxygenation. J Leukoc Biol 65:171–178
29. Guillemin K and Krasnow MA (1997) The hypoxic response: Huffing and HIFing. Cell 89:9–12
30. Guleng B, Tateishi K, Ohta M, et al. (2005) Blockade of the stromal cell derived factor-1 / CXCR4 axis attenuates *in vivo* tumor growth by inhibiting angiogenesis in vascular endothelial growth factor-independent manner. Cancer Res 13:5864–5871
31. Hanahan D and Folkman J (1996) Patterns and emerging mechanism of the angiogenic switch during tumorigenesis. Cell 86:353–364
32. Hendrix CW, Collier AC, Lederman MM, et al. (2004) Safety, pharmacokinetics, and antiviral activity of AMD3100, a selective CXCR4 receptor inhibitor, in HIV-1 infection. J Acquir Immune Defic Syndr 37:1253–1262
33. Hong X, Jiang F, Kalkanis SN, et al. (2006) SDF-1 and CXCR4 are up-regulated by VEGF and contribute to glioma cell invasion. Cancer Letts 236:39–45
34. Huang LE, Arany Z, Livingston DM, et al. (1996) Activation of hypoxia-inducible transcription factor depends primarily upon redox-sensitive stabilization of its alpha subunit. J Biol Chem 271:32253–32259
35. Huang LE, Gu J, Schau M, et al. (1998) Regulation of hypoxia-inducible factor 1alpha is mediated by an O2-dependent degradation domain via the ubiquitin-proteasome pathway. Proc Natl Acad Sci USA 95:7987–7992

36. Jiang BH., Semenza GL, Bauer C, et al. (1996) Hypoxia-inducible factor 1 levels vary exponentially over a physiologically relevant range of O2 tension. Am J Physiol 271: C1172-C1180
37. Jung YJ, Isaacs JS, Lee S, et al. (2003) IL-1beta-mediated up-regulation of HIF-1alpha via an NFkappaB/COX-2 pathway identifies HIF-1 as a critical link between inflammation and oncogenesis. FASEB J 17:2115–2117
38. Kallio PJ, Wilson WJ, O'Brien S, et al. (1999) Regulation of the hypoxia-inducible transcription factor 1alpha by the ubiquitin-proteasome pathway. J Biol Chem 274: 6519–6525
39. Kim SY, Lee CH, Midura BV, et al. (2007) Inhibition of the CXCR4/CXCL12 chemokine pathway reduces the development of murine pulmonary metastases. Clin Exp Metastasis DOI 10.1007/s10585-007-9133-3
40. Kodama J, Hasengaowa L, Kusomoto T, et al. (2007) Association of CXCR4 and CCR7 chemokine receptor expression and lymph node metastasis in human cervical cancer. Ann Oncol 18:70–76
41. Kopp HG, Ramos CA, Rafii S (2006) Contribution of endothelial progenitors and proangiogenic hematopoietic cells to vascularization of tumor and ischemic tissue. Curr Opin Hematol 13:175–181
42. Krishnamachary B, Berg-Dixon S, Kelly B, et al. (2003) Regulation of colon carcinoma cell invasion by hypoxia-inducible factor 1. Cancer Res 63:1138–1143
43. Kryczek I, Wei S, Keller E, et al. (2007) Stromal-derived factor (SDF-1/CXCL12) and human pathogenesis. Am J Physiol Cell Physiol 292:C987-C995
44. Kucia M, Reca R, Miekus K, et al. (2005) Trafficking of normal stem cells and metastasis of cancer stem cells involve similar mechanisms: Pivotal role of the SDF-1-CXCR4 axis. Stem Cells 23:879–894
45. Kulbe H, Levinson NR, Balkwill F, et al. (2004) The chemokine network in cancer – much more than directing cell movement. Int J Dev Biol 48:489–496
46. Lakka SS, Gondi CS, Dinh DH, et al. (2005) Specific interference of urokinase-type plasminogen activator receptor and matrix metalloproteinase-9 gene expression induced by double-stranded RNA results in decreased invasion, tumor growth, and angiogenesis in gliomas. J Biol Chem 280:21882–21892
47. Li M and Ransohoff RM (2008) Multiple roles of chemokine CXCL12 in the central nervous system: A migration from immunology to neurobiology. Prog Neurobiol 84:116–131
48. Liang Z, Wu T, Lou H, et al. (2004) Inhibition of breast cancer metastasis by selective synthetic polypeptide against CXCR4. Cancer Res 64:4302–4308
49. Liang Z, Yoon Y, Votaw J, et al. (2005) Silencing of CXCR4 blocks breast cancer metastasis. Cancer Res 65:967–971
50. Maxwell PJ, Gallagher R, Seaton A, et al. (2007) HIF-1 and NF-kappaB-mediated upregulation of CXCR1 and CXCR2 expression promotes cell survival in hypoxic prostate cancer cells. Oncogene 26:7333–7345
51. Miao Z, Luker KE, Summers BC, et al. (2007) CXCR7 (RDC1) promotes breast and lung tumor growth in vivo and is expressed on tumor-associated vasculature. Proc Natl Acad Sci USA 104:15735–15740
52. Mizukami Y, Jo WS, Duerr EM, et al. (2005) Induction of interleukin-8 preserves the angiogenic response in HIF-1alpha-deficient colon cancer cells. Nat Med 11:992–997
53. Mizukami Y, Kohgo Y, Chung DC (2007) Hypoxia inducible factor-1- independent pathways in tumor angiogenesis. Clin Cancer Res 13:5670–5674
54. Moldobaeva A and Wagner EM (2005) Difference in proangiogenic potential of systemic and pulmonary endothelium: Role of CXCR2. Am J Physiol Lung Cell Mol Physiol 288:L1117–1123
55. Muller A, Sonkoly E, Eulert C, et al. (2005) Chemokine receptors in head and neck cancer: Association with metastatic spread and regulation during chemotherapy. Int J Cancer 118:2147–2157

56. Murphy C, McGurk M, Pettigrew J, et al. (2005) Nonapical and cytoplasmic expression of interleukin-8, CXCR1, and CXCR2 correlates with cell proliferation and microvessel density in prostate cancer. Clin Cancer Res 11:4117–4127
57. Oda Y, Yamamoto H, Tamiya S, et al. (2006) CXCR4 and VEGF expression in the primary site and the metastatic site of human osteosarcoma: Analysis within a group of patients, all of whom developed lung metastasis. Mod Pathol 19:738–745
58. Oh JW, Drabik K, Kutsch O, et al. (2001) CXC chemokine receptor 4 expression and function in human astroglioma cells. J Immunol 166:2695–2704
59. Ottaiano A, Franco R, Talamanca AA, et al. (2006) Overexpression of both CXC chemokine receptor 4 and vascular endothelial growth factor proteins predicts early distant relapse in stage II-III colorectal cancer patients. Clin Cancer Res 12:2795–2799
60. Ou DL, Chen CL, Lin SB, et al. (2006) Chemokine receptor expression profiles in nasopharyngeal carcinoma and their association with metastasis and radiotherapy. J Pathol 210:363–373
61. Pan J, Mestas J, Burdick M, et al. (2006) Stromal cell derived factor -1 (SDF-1/CXCL12) and CXCR4 in renal cell carcinoma metastasis. Mol Cancer DOI:10.1186/1476-4598-5-56
62. Petit I, Jin D, Rafii S (2007) The SDF-1-CXCR4 signaling pathway: A molecular hub modulating neo-angiogenesis. Trends Immunol 28:299–307
63. Piovan E, Tosello V, Indraccolo S, et al. (2007) Differential regulation of hypoxia-induced CXCR4 triggering during B-cell development and lymphomagenesis. Cancer Res 67:8605–8614
64. Plasswilm L, Tannapfel A, Cordes N, et al. (2000) Hypoxia-induced tumour cell migra- tion in an in vivo chicken model. Pathobiology 2000; 68:99–105
65. Ratajczak MZ, Zuba-Surma E, Kucia M, et al. (2006) The pleiotropic effects of the SDF-1-CXCR4 axis in organogenesis, regeneration and tumorigenesis. Leukemia 20: 1915–1924
66. Redjal N, Chan JA, Segal RA, et al. (2006) CXCR4 inhibition synergizes with cytotoxic chemotherapy in gliomas. Clin Cancer Res 12:6765–6771
67. Rempel SA, Dudas S, Ge S, et al. (2000) Identification and localization of the cytokine SDF1 and its receptor, CXC chemokine receptor 4, to regions of necrosis and angiogen- esis in human glioblastoma. Clin Cancer Res 6:102–111
68. Retz M, Sidhu S, Blaveri E, et al. (2005) CXCR4 expression reflects tumor progression and regulates motility of bladder cancer cells. Int J Cancer 114:182–189
69. Rubin JB, Kung AL, Klein RS, et al. (2003) A small-molecule antagonist of CXCR4 inhibits intracranial growth of primary brain tumors. Proc Natl Acad Sci USA 100:13513–13518
70. Ruffini PA, Morandi P, Cabioglu N, et al. (2007) Manipulating the chemokine-chemokine receptor network to treat cancer. Cancer 109:2392–2404
71. Russell H, Hicks J, Okcu F, et al. (2004) CXCR4 expression in neuroblastoma primary tumors is associated with clinical presentation of bone and bone marrow metastases. J Pediat Surg 39:1503–1511
72. Salceda S and Caro J (1997) Hypoxia-inducible factor 1alpha (HIF-1alpha) protein is rapidly degraded by the ubiquitin-proteasome system under normoxic conditions. Its stabilization by hypoxia depends on redox-induced changes. J Biol Chem 272: 22642–22647
73. Schimanski C, Bahre R, Gockel I, et al. (2006) Dissemination of hepatocellular carci- noma is mediated via chemokine receptor CXCR4. B J Cancer 95:210–217
74. Schioppa T, Uranchimeg B, Saccani A, et al. (2003) Regulation of the chemokine CXCR4 by hypoxia. J Exp Med 198:1391–1402
75. Schutyser E, Su Y, Yu Y, et al. (2007) Hypoxia enhances CXCR4 expression in human microvascular endothelial cells and human melanoma cells. Eur Cytokine Netw 18:59–70
76. Semenza GL (1999) Regulation of mammalian O2 homeostasis by hypoxia-inducible factor 1. Annu Rev Cell Dev Biol 15:551–578

77. Semenza GL (2003) Targeting HIF-1 for cancer therapy. Nat Rev Cancer 3:721–732
78. Semenza GL (2007) Hypoxia-inducible factor 1 (HIF-1) pathway. Sci STKE 407:cm8-cm12.
79. Serratí S, Margheri F, Fibbi G, et al. (2008) Endothelial cells and normal breast epithelial cells enhance invasion of breast carcinoma cells by CXCR-4-dependent up-regulation of urokinase-type plasminogen activator receptor (uPAR, CD87) expression. J Pathol 214:545–554
80. Shim H, Lau SK, Devi S, et al. (2006) Lower expression of CXCR4 in lymph node metastases than in primary breast cancers: Potential regulation by ligand-dependent degradation and HIF-1α. Biochem Biophys Res Commun 346:252–258
81. Singh S, Singh UP, Grizzle WE, et al. (2004) CXCL12-CXCR4 interactions modulate prostate cancer cell migration, metalloproteinase expression and invasion. Lab Invest 84:1666–1676
82. Spring H, Schuler T, Arnold B, et al. (2005) Chemokines direct endothelial progenitors into tumor neovessels. Proc Natl Acad Sci USA 102:18111–18116
83. Staller P, Sulitkova J, Lisztwan J, et al. (2003) Chemokine receptor CXCR4 downregulated by Hippel-Lindau tumour suppressor pVHL. Nature 425;307–311
84. Steeg PS (2003) Angiogenesis inhibitors: Motivators of metastasis? Nat Med 9:822–823
85. Strahm B, Durbin A, Sexsmith E, et al. (2008) The CXCR4-SDF1α axis is a critical mediator of rhabdomyosarcoma metastatic signaling induced by bone marrow stroma. Clin Exp Metastasis 25:1–10
86. Strieter RM, Polverini PJ, Kunkel SL, et al. (1995) The functional role of the ELR motif in CXC chemokine-mediated angiogenesis. J Biol Chem 270:27348–27357
87. Struckmann K, Mertz K, Steu S, et al. (2008) pVHL co-ordinately regulates CXCR4/CXCL12 and MMP2/MMP9 expression in human clear-cell renal cell carcinoma. J Pathol 214:463–471
88. Su L, Zhang J, Xu H, et al. (2005) Differential expression of CXCR4 is associated with the metastatic potential of human non-small lung cancer cells. Clin Cancer Res 23:8273–8280
89. Szekanecz Z and Koch AE (2007) Mechanisms of disease: Angiogenesis in inflammatory diseases. Nat Clin Pract Rheumatol 3:635–643
90. Trentin L, Miorin M, Facco M, et al. (2007) Multiple myeloma plasma cells show different chemokine receptor profiles at sites of disease activity. Br J Haematol 138:594–602
91. Tucci MG, Lucarini G, Brancorsini D, et al. (2007) Involvement of E-cadherin, β-catenin, Cdc42 and CXCR4 in the progression and prognosis of cutaneous melanoma. Br J Dermatol 157:1212–1216
92. Uchida D, Onoue T, Tomizuka Y, et al. (2007) Involvement of an autocrine stromal cell derived factor-1/CXCR4 system on the distant metastasis of human oral squamous cell carcinoma. Mol Cancer Res 7:685–694
93. Wang GL, Jiang BH, Rue EA, et al. (1995) Hypoxia-inducible factor 1 is a basic-helix-loop-helix-PAS heterodimer regulated by cellular O2 tension. Proc Natl Acad Sci USA 92:5510–5514
94. Wang J, Shiozawa Y, Wang J, et al. (2008) The role of CXCR7/RDC1 as a chemokine receptor for CXCL12/SDF-1 in prostate cancer. J Biol Chem 283:4283–4294
95. Warner KA, Miyazawa M, Cordeiro MM, et al. (2008) Endothelial cells enhance tumor cell invasion through a crosstalk mediated by CXC chemokine signaling. Neoplasia 10:131–139
96. Wehler T, Wolfert F, Schimanski C, et al. (2006) Strong expression of chemokine receptor = CXCR4 by pancreatic cancer correlates with advanced disease. Oncol Rep 16:1159–1164
97. Woerner BM, Warrington NM, Kung AL, et al. (2005) Widespread CXCR4 activation in astrocytomas revealed by phospho-CXCR4-specific antibodies. Cancer Res 65:11392–11399

98. Woo S, Bae J, Kim C, et al. (2007) A significant correlation between nuclear CXCR4 expression and axillary lymph node metastasis in hormonal receptor negative breast cancer. Ann Surg Oncol 15:281–285
99. Xie K (2001) Interleukin-8 and human cancer biology. Cytokine Growth Factor Rev 12:375–391
100. Yang L, Jackson E, Woerner BM, et al. (2007a) Blocking CXCR4-mediated cyclic AMP suppression inhibits brain tumor growth in vivo. Cancer Res 67:651–658
101. Yang YC, Lee ZY, Wu CC, et al. (2007b) CXCR4 expression is associated with pelvic lymph node metastasis in cervical adenocarcinoma. Int J Gynecol Cancer 17:676–686
102. Yasumoto K, Koizumi K, Kawashima A, et al. (2006) Role of CXCL12/CXCR4 axis in peritoneal carcinomatosis of gastric cancer. Cancer Res 4:2181–2187
103. Yoon Y, Liang Z, Zhang X, et al. (2007) CXC chemokine receptor-4 antagonist blocks both growth of primary tumor and metastasis of head and neck cancer in xenograft mouse models. Cancer Res 15:7518–7524
104. Zagzag D, Zhong H, Scalzitti JM, et al. (2000) Expression of hypoxia-inducible factor 1alpha in brain tumors: Association with angiogenesis, invasion, and progression. Cancer 88:2606–2618
105. Zagzag D, Krishnamachary B, Yee H, et al. (2005) Stromal cell-derived factor-1α and CXCR4 expression in hemangioblastomas and clear cell-renal cell carcinoma: von Hippel-Lindau loss-of-function induces expression of a ligand and its receptor. Cancer Res 65:6178–6188
106. Zagzag D, Lukyanov Y, Lan L, et al. (2006) Hypoxia-inducible factor 1 and VEGF upregulate CXCR4 in glioblastoma: Implications for angiogenesis and glioma cell invasion. Lab Invest 86:1221–1232
107. Zagzag D, Esencay M, Mendez O, et al. (2008) Hypoxia- and vascular endothelial growth factor-induced stromal cell-derived factor-1alpha/CXCR4 expression in glioblastomas: One plausible explanation of Scherer's structures. Am J Pathol 173:545–560
108. Zhang J, Lu W, Ye F, et al. (2007) Study on CXCR4/SDF-1 axis in lymph node metastasis of cervical squamous cell carcinoma. Int J Gynecol Cancer 17:478–483
109. Zhang J, Sarkar S, Yong VW (2005) The chemokine stromal cell derived factor-1 (CXCL12) promotes glioma invasiveness through MT2-matrix metalloproteinase. Carcinogenesis 26:2069–2077
110. Zhou Y, Larsen PH, Hao C, et al. (2002) CXCR4 is a major chemokine receptor on glioma cells and mediates their survival. J Biol Chem 277:49481–49487
111. Zhong H, De Marzo AM, Laughner E, et al. (1999) Overexpression of hypoxia-inducible factor-1α in common human cancers and their metastases. Cancer Res 59:5830–5835
112. Zhu YM, Bagstaff SM, Woll PJ (2006) Production and upregulation of granulocyte chemotactic protien-2/CXCL6 by IL-1b and hypoxia in small cell lung cancer. Br J Cancer 94:1936–1941
113. Zlotnik A and Yoshie O (2000) Chemokines a new classification system and their role in immunity. Immunity 12:121–127
114. Zlotnik A (2004) Chemokines in neoplastic progression. Sem Cancer Biol 14:181–185
115. Zlotnik A (2008) New insights on the role of CXCR4 in cancer metastasis. J Pathol 215:211–213

Chemokine Receptors Involved in Colon Cancer Progression, and Lymph Node Metastasis

Makoto Mark Taketo and Kenji Kawada

Abstract In this chapter, we focus on the roles of chemokines and their receptors on colon cancer invasion, and lymph node metastasis in two mouse models. First, inactivation of TGF-β family signaling within colon cancer epithelium increases chemokine CCL9, and promotes recruitment of the MMP-expressing stromal cells that carry CCR1, the cognate receptor for CCL9. Consistently, lack of CCR1 prevents the accumulation of MMP-expressing myeloid cells at the invasion front and suppresses tumor invasion. These results provide the possibility of a novel therapeutic strategy for advanced cancer; prevention of the recruitment of MMP-expressing myeloid cells by chemokine receptor antagonist; hence "cellular target therapy" instead of molecular target therapy. Second, we recently found that some human colon cancer cell lines express chemokine receptor CXCR3 constitutively. To evaluate its role in metastasis, we constructed colon cancer cells that expressed CXCR3 cDNA (DLD-1-CXCR3), and compared with non-expressing controls by rectal transplantation in nude mice. In 6 weeks, 59% of mice inoculated with DLD1-CXCR3 showed macroscopic metastasis in para-aortic lymph nodes, whereas only 14% of those with the control ($P < 0.05$). Metastasis to the liver or lung was rare, and unaffected by CXCR3 expression. In human colon cancer specimens, expression of CXCR3 was found in 34% cases, most of which had lymph node metastasis. Importantly, patients with CXCR3-positive colon cancer showed significantly poorer prognosis than those without CXCR3, or those expressing CXCR4 or CCR7. These results indicate that activation of CXCR3 stimulates colon cancer metastasis preferentially to the draining lymph nodes with poorer prognosis.

M.M. Taketo (✉)
Department of Pharmacology, Graduate School of Medicine, Kyoto University,
Sakyo, Kyoto 606-8501, Japan
e-mail: taketo@mfour.med.kyoto-u.ac.jp

A.M. Fulton (ed.), *Chemokine Receptors in Cancer*, Cancer Drug Discovery
and Development, DOI 10.1007/978-1-60327-267-4_4,
© Humana Press, a part of Springer Science+Business Media, LLC 2009

63

Chemokines and Their Receptors in Cancer

Chemokines are chemotactic cytokines that direct the migration of chemokine receptor-expressing cells. They are structurally related, small polypeptide signaling molecules that bind to, and activate a family of G-protein-coupled receptors. Chemokines are divided into four families: CXC, CC, C, and CX_3C, based on the positions of four conserved cysteine residues. Important roles of chemokines and their receptors have been demonstrated in inflammation, infection, tissue injury, allergy, and cardiovascular diseases, as well as in malignant tumors [6]. Although originally identified for leukocyte trafficking in infections, the chemokine–chemokine receptor system plays complex roles in tumors. Whereas many chemokines show anti-tumor activity by stimulating immune cells or by inhibiting tumor neovascularization, other chemokines may promote tumor growth and metastasis by direct growth stimulation, enhancing cell motility or angiogenesis [55]. For example, tumor cells from various types of cancer carry chemokine receptor CXCR4 and metastasize to the bone and lung, where its ligand CXCL12 is expressed [24, 35]. In this chapter, we focus on the roles of chemokines and their receptors on colon cancer invasion, and lymph node metastasis.

Genetic Changes in Colon Cancer Progression and Stromal Reactions

Colorectal cancer develops progressively through accumulation of genetic lesions in the epithelial cells. Namely, most adenomas are initiated by inactivation of the *APC* gene in the colonic epithelial cells, and progress into malignant adenocarcinomas through accumulation of additional genetic alterations in the *KRAS*, p53 (*TP53*), *SMAD4*, and TGF-β receptor type II (*TGFBR2*) genes, etc. [56]. While these genetic lesions can contribute to tumor progression through increased proliferation and decreased apoptosis in the tumor cells, genetic mechanisms that are responsible for adenocarcinoma metastasis are only beginning to be unraveled.

In addition to these cell-autonomous changes in the epithelial compartment, it is becoming clear that the stromal cells surrounding the tumor epithelium play key roles in the development of various types of cancer. In addition to the essential roles of angiogenesis in tumor stroma [23], tumor-infiltrating leukocytes contribute to skin carcinogenesis [7], and cancer-associated fibroblasts (CAFs) stimulate prostate tumor formation [37]. CAFs also promote the growth of breast cancer xenografts [38]. Furthermore, depletion of tumor-associated macrophages reduces metastasis in a breast cancer mouse model [32], suggesting that the stromal cells affect not only tumor initiation and growth, but also metastasis. More recently, it has been demonstrated that the mesenchymal stem cells also play a role in breast cancer metastasis [25]. However, precise roles of the stromal cells in cancer invasion, apparently the first step in metastasis, were not understood thoroughly until recently. It also remained unclear how genetic lesions in the tumor epithelial cells, such as inactivation of the *SMAD4* or *TGFBR2* genes, lead to stromal cell accumulation and activation.

Tumor-Stromal Interaction in Colon Cancer Invasion: A Mouse Model

As a model of colorectal tumor progression, we earlier constructed compound mutant mouse strain " *cis-Apc/Smad4*" that carried homozygous inactivation of both *Apc* and *Smad4* genes specifically in the tumor epithelium [48]. The *cis-Apc/Smad4* mice develop intestinal adenocarcinomas that show marked invasion, in contrast to the simple $Apc^{+/-}$ (i.e., $Apc^{+/\Delta716}$) mutant mice that develop only benign adenomas. Like most epithelial cancers, the *cis-Apc/Smad4* adenocarcinomas invade the intestinal wall as protruding glands or sheets, a typical pattern of "collective migration" [14]. This type of invasion is assumed as an early stage of epithelial tumor metastasis because tumor collectives or clusters can be detected in the circulation of patients with adenocarcinomas.

In a recent study, we found that the invading tumor glands of the *cis-Apc/Smad4* adenocarcinomas were associated with clusters of "immature myeloid cells (iMCs)" that expressed myeloid progenitor cell marker CD34, pan-leukocyte marker CD45, and myeloid cell marker CD11b [29]. To examine the mechanism underlying the accumulation of these cells, we looked for chemokines that were increased in the *cis-Apc/Smad4* polyps because chemokines stimulate directed cell movement (see below). Among the chemokines tested, only CC-chemokine ligand 9 (CCL9) was increased significantly in the *cis-Apc/Smad4* tumor epithelium. Because the *Smad4* genes are lost only in the tumor epithelial cells, as defined by the genetic design of the *cis-Apc/Smad4* mice [29, 48], these results indicate that loss of the TGF-β family signaling in the tumor epithelium can promote the production of chemokine CCL9. Consistently, we found that expression of CCL9 in mouse colon cancer cell line CT26 was suppressed by TGF-β family ligands such as TGF-β, activin, BMP4, and BMP7. We further examined expression of CC-chemokine receptor 1 (CCR1), the cognate receptor for CCL9, and found that the CD34$^+$ immature myeloid cells at the invasion front express CCR1 and migrate toward the ligand CCL9.

We then assessed the role of CCR1 in recruiting CD34$^+$ immature myeloid cells toward the polyps. To this end, we introduced a homozygous *Ccr1* knockout mutation into the *cis-Apc/Smad4* mice and found that lack of CCR1 prevents the accumulation of immature myeloid cells at the invasion front. Importantly, the loss of CCR1 dramatically suppressed tumor invasion into the smooth muscle layer and serosa in the *cis-Apc/Smad4* mice. Because immature myeloid cells at the invasion front showed gelatinolytic activities and expressed matrix metalloproteinase (MMP) 9 and 2, these results indicate that the immature myeloid cells help tumor invasion, at least in part through the production of MMPs.

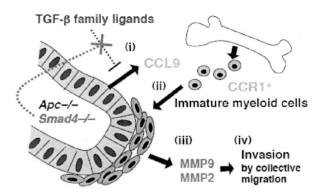

Fig. 1 SMAD4-deficient tumor cells produce chemokine CCL9 and recruit the receptor-expressing cells that promote tumor invasion in early stages. The inactivation of the TGF-β family signaling within the tumor epithelium causes increased production of chemokine CCL9 because it is suppressed by TGF-β, activin-A and BMPs (i). Increased levels of CCL9 recruit immature myeloid cells that carry the CCL9 receptor CCR1 from the blood to the tumor invasion front (ii). These immature myeloid cells produce MMP9 and 2 (iii), and help the tumor epithelium to migrate and invade into the stroma *en masse* (iv). Reproduced with permission from Kitamura, T. and Taketo, M.M. (2007) Keeping out bad guys: Gateway to the cellular target therapy. *Cancer Res,* **2007,** 1009–10102

Taken together, our recent findings indicate that loss of TGF-β family signaling within tumor epithelium stimulates chemokine CCL9 secretion, which results in the accumulation of immature myeloid cells that help tumor invasion (Fig. 1).

From "Molecular Target" Therapy to "Cellular Target" Therapy

As described above, lack of CCR1 prevented the accumulation of MMP-expressing cells at the invasion front and suppressed tumor invasion in the *cis-Apc/Smad4* mice. Similar to the *cis-Apc/Smad4* polyps, the CCR1$^+$ cells that expressed MMP9 infiltrated at the invasion front of some human colon cancers with *TGFBR2* mutations [29], suggesting the key roles of the stromal cells that express MMPs in invasion. Accordingly, these results provide a novel strategy for cancer therapy that targets the "assisting stromal cells", using chemokine receptor antagonists to prevent accumulation of the MMP-expressing cells.

Because MMPs degrade the extracellular matrix (ECM) that separates tumor epithelium from the initially normal stroma, they contribute to the tumor invasion and subsequent metastasis. Consistent with this notion, many clinical studies of colon cancer have shown that expression levels of MMP2 and MMP9 correlate with tumor progression [34]. However, attempts to block MMPs directly to prevent tumor progression have failed in the extensive phase III clinical trials. Almost all MMP inhibitors from multiple companies could not show clinical efficiency. Even worse, some compounds had severe side effects such as inflammation, musculoskeletal pain, and joint strictures [40].

In retrospect, the attempts to inhibit MMPs failed because they cleave not only ECM components, but also many other proteins including growth factor-binding proteins, cytokine precursors, chemokines, etc. [40]. The proteolysis of these MMP substrates results in the release and/or activation of secreted factors that stimulate stomal cell infiltration and proliferation. Therefore, it is not surprising that systemic and prolonged inhibition of MMP activities causes aberrant immune responses and other stromal reactions. The ineffectiveness of MMP inhibitors may be explained partly by the recent findings that cancer stromal cells have non-MMP proteases that degrade ECM, such as cathepsins [16] and uPARAP/Endo 180 [8].

Compared with the systemic "molecular target" therapy using MMP inhibitors, the "cellular target" therapy using CCR1 antagonists may cause much less side effects because chemokines affect only tissue-specific and therefore localized cell migration. Consistently, a mouse study indicates that the effect of CCR1 deficiency is rather benign unless the mice are infected [15]. Instead of direct and systemic inhibition of MMPs, the blockade of MMP-producing cell accumulation by CCR1 antagonists might help improve management of some advanced tumors.

CCR1 Antagonists

It has been reported that CCR1 binds several chemokines including CCL3, CCL5, CCL7, as well as CCL9, and is associated with various autoimmune diseases such as multiple sclerosis, rheumatoid arthritis, organ-transplant rejection, etc. [19]. Therefore, some pharmaceutical companies have developed CCR1 antagonists, and are testing some compounds in phase II clinical trials for multiple sclerosis and rheumatoid arthritis [19].

Among the reported CCR1 antagonists, one of the well-characterized compounds appears to be BX471 developed by Berlex. In competitive binding assays, BX471 inhibits in a dose-dependent manner the binding of CCL3, CCL5, and CCL7 to human CCR1 with Ki values of 2.8, 1.0, and 5.5 nM, respectively [19]. Furthermore, BX471 suppresses human leukocyte migration stimulated by the CCR1 ligands, but not those by ligands of CCR2, CCR5, or CXCR4, suggesting that it is a functional antagonist with selective specificity to CCR1. Using animal models of autoimmune diseases, many reports suggest the efficacy of this compound as a therapeutic. Namely, BX471 reduces a clinical score in a rat experimental allergic encephalomyelitis model of multiple sclerosis [31], and blocks rat heart transplant rejection in combination with cyclosporine [20]. Because some CCR1 antagonists including BX471 have already been tested for their safety, we can advocate these compounds as potential drug candidates for colon cancer progression.

Chemokine Receptor CXCR3 and Lymph Node Metastasis

Chemokine receptor CXCR3 is essential for the physiologic and pathologic recruitment of plasmacytoid dendritic cell precursors, monocytes, and natural killer cells to inflamed lymph nodes (LNs) [3, 21, 33], and for retention of Th1 lymphocytes within LNs [58]. On the other hand, chemokine receptor CCR7 plays a central role in the recruitment of naïve T cells, some memory T cells, and mature dendritic cells to LNs [9, 53]. Regarding the direct role of chemokines in LN metastasis, recent reports suggest a critical role for chemokine receptors CXCR3 and CCR7 in metastasis of melanoma and breast cancer [27, 35, 45]. Importantly, both CXCR3 and CCR7 are involved in the recruitment and patterning of several types of immune cells to the LNs, suggesting that tumor cells have acquired these receptors and are controlled by their ligands in a manner analogous to the immune cell interactions.

Concerning the expression of CXCR3 ligands in various normal organs, we found that the mRNA levels for CXCL9, CXCL10, and CCL21 were expressed preferentially in lymphoid organs such as LNs and spleen, but not in the liver, lung, large intestine, or skin, although a low level of CXCL9 was found in the liver. In contrast, CXCL11 was hardly expressed in any of these organs. We further examined expression and localization of CXCL9, CXCL10, and CCL21 proteins within LNs by immunohistochemistry, and found that both CXCL9 and CXCL10 were expressed mainly in the subcapsular and cortical sinuses, and CCL21 throughout the T zone.

We earlier demonstrated that CXCR3 expressed on melanoma cells plays a critical role in their metastasis from the foot pads to popliteal LNs [27]. We constructed B16F10 melanoma cells with reduced CXCR3 expression by anti-sense RNA and investigated their metastatic activities after subcutaneous (s.c.) inoculations into the foot pads. The metastatic frequency of these cells to popliteal LNs was markedly reduced compared with the control cells. On the other hand, pretreatment with complete Freund's adjuvant increased the levels of CXCR3 ligands in the popliteal LNs, which caused a significant increase in the metastatic frequency to popliteal LNs. Importantly, such a stimulation of metastasis was largely suppressed when CXCR3 expression in B16F10 cells was reduced by antisense RNA or when mice were treated with specific antibodies against CXCL9 and CXCL10.

Expression of CXCR3 in Colon Cancer Cell Lines

To determine the roles of CXCR3 in colon cancer metastasis, we first examined expression of chemokine receptors (CXCR3, CXCR4, and CCR7) in human colon cancer cell lines, and found that CXCR3 was expressed constitutively at high levels in five (Colo205, HCT116, HT29, RKO, and WiDr) of ten cell lines. In addition, we found that CCR7 was expressed only in two (SW480 and

Caco2) cell lines, whereas CXCR4 was detected in seven cell lines (Colo205, HCT116, HT29, WiDr, SW480, LS174T, and Caco2).

In addition to CXCL9, CXCL10, and CXCL11, it has been reported that a ligand for CCR7, CCL21/SLC can also bind to and activate CXCR3 in mice [47]. Also in some human cells, CCL21 is a functional ligand for endogenously expressed CXCR3 [10, 42]. Addition of CXCL10 and CXCL12 to Colo205 that expressed CXCR3 and CXCR4 but not CCR7, induced cell migration, and a neutralizing anti-CXCR3 antibody significantly suppressed the migratory response in a dose-dependent manner. In addition, Colo205 cells exhibit CCL21-induced migration with a little lower efficiency than CXCL10, which indicates that CCL21 induces chemotaxis of human colon cancer cell line Colo205 through CXCR3. Regarding the cell growth and survival, neither CXCL10 nor CCL21 had any effects on cell proliferation under the normal (10% FCS) or low (0.5% FCS) serum condition. Without serum, however, both ligands significantly enhanced cell survival, compared with the untreated controls. Tumor cells often encounter stress conditions, hypoxia, immune responses, or nutrient deprivation. Accordingly, we investigated regulation of CXCR3 in colon cancer cells under stress by serum deprivation. The total cellular protein levels of CXCR3 were similar between high serum (10% FCS) and serum-starved cultures for 3 days. However, expression of CXCR3 on the membrane changed dramatically upon serum starvation. Namely, most cells in the population expressed CXCR3 in the absence of serum, whereas only approximately half did in its presence, although total cellular receptor content remained at similar levels. Thus, it is possible that expression of CXCR3 on the cell surface helps tumor cells to survive under stress. Concerning MMPs, expression and activities of MMP2 and MMP9 were significantly increased by addition of CXCL10, which was suppressed by CXCR3 neutralization.

Enhanced Metastasis of DLD-1-CXCR3 Cells to Draining Lymph Nodes

To investigate whether CXCR3 plays a role in colon cancer metastasis, we introduced a retroviral expression vector for CXCR3 into DLD-1 cells that expressed neither CXCR3 nor CCR7 (Fig. 2A). In this construct, CXCR3 mRNA was expressed from an LTR promoter followed by an internal ribosome entry site (IRES) and enhanced GFP (EGFP) cDNA. Although the transduction efficiency was approximately 10%, we could sort by FACS the cell population that expressed EGFP efficiently ("DLD-1-CXCR3" cells). We also isolated cells expressing an empty vector that contained EGFP, but not CXCR3 ("DLD-1-EV" cells).

The rectal xenograft method offers a convenient animal model for colorectal cancer that can metastasize to the draining para-aortic LNs [26, 36, 51]. To assess the effect of CXCR3 expression on LN metastasis, we inoculated

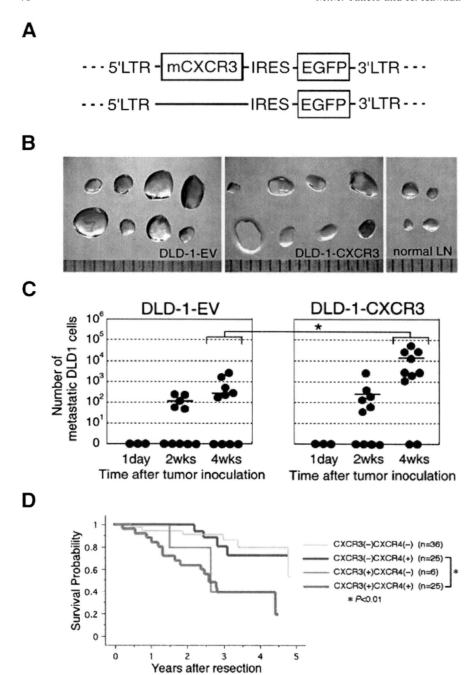

Fig. 2 Stimulation of colon cancer cell metastasis to LNs by expression of CXCR3. (**A**) Partial structures are shown for the construct (*top*), and empty vector pMX-IRES-EGFP used as the

DLD-1-CXCR3 and DLD-1-EV cells, respectively, in the rectum of nude mice. One week later, transplanted rectal tumors became grossly visible, and their size increased rapidly with time. Six weeks later, we examined macroscopically metastatic foci of the para-aortic LNs using GFP fluorescence. Under a fluorescence dissection microscope, we found that DLD-1-CXCR3 cells metastasized to LNs with a significantly higher frequency than DLD-1-EV (Fig. 2B). Although 14% (3 of 22) of the mice inoculated with DLD-1-EV cells showed visible metastatic foci of relatively small size, 59% (13 of 22) of the mice with DLD-1-CXCR3 formed larger foci ($P < 0.01$). Regarding the transplanted primary rectal tumors, there was no significant difference in size between the two groups. As for metastasis to the lung or liver, there was no significant difference between the two groups.

To quantify the metastasized DLD-1 cells to the para-aortic LNs, we determined the level of human β-globin related sequence (HBB) by quantitative PCR (Fig. 2C). One day after inoculation, we detected no amplified signals from LNs. Two weeks later, we found DNA of DLD-1-EV and DLD-1-CXCR3 cells in LNs in 5 of 10, and 6 of 10 mice, respectively. The number of cells spread to LNs was estimated to be ≤ 500/mouse, except one mouse with DLD-1-CXCR3 cells. The result indicated that there was no apparent difference in the number of DLD-1 cells disseminated to LNs between the two groups at this stage (DLD-1-EV, 120 ± 90 cells; and DLD-1-CXCR3, 510 ± 1200 cells; mean $\pm$ SD of 10 transplants/group). Four weeks after inoculations, we occasionally found GFP fluorescence from DLD-1-CXCR3 foci in the LNs, although we never found such foci in mice inoculated with DLD-1-EV. Quantification of metastasized DLD-1 cells showed that the number of DLD-1-CXCR3 cells in LNs was significantly higher than that of DLD-1-EV (DLD-1-EV, $\sim 500 \pm 700$ cells; and DLD-1-CXCR3, $20,000 \pm 28,000$ cells; mean $\pm$ SD of 10 transplants/group) (Fig. 2C; $P < 0.05$). These results suggest that activation of CXCR3 is important for establishing metastatic foci of colon cancer cells in LNs.

Fig. 2 (continued) negative control (*bottom*). (**B**) Representative photographs of the para-aortic LNs from mice 6 weeks after inoculations with DLD-1-EV (*left*) and DLD-1-CXCR3 (*center*) cells, respectively. Normal LNs from uninoculated control mice are also shown (*right*). Metastatic foci are visualized by GFP fluorescence. Scale in mm. (**C**) Time course of the tumor cell metastasis in LNs. Ten mice from each group were analyzed at the indicated time after tumor inoculation. The para-aortic LNs were pooled for each mouse and extracted DNA was analyzed for the numbers of metastasized tumor cells using the human β-globin gene (HBB). The estimation was based on a calibration curve of given numbers of cultured DLD-1 cells. Mean; bars (*, $P < 0.05$ by Student's t-test). (**D**) Survival curves (Kaplan and Meier estimates) by expression of CXCR3 and CXCR4 in colon cancer. Reproduced with permission from Kawada, K., Hosogi, H., Sonoshita, M., et al. (2007) Chemokine receptor CXCR3 promotes colon cancer metastasis to lymph nodes. *Oncogene*, **26**, 4679–4688

CXCR3 Expression in Clinical Colon Cancer Samples

To evaluate the clinical relevance of the above results, we immunohistochemically examined specimens from 92 colon cancer patients for expression of CXCR3 and CCR7 as well as CXCR4. We found that 31 samples (33.7%) expressed CXCR3 in cancer epithelial cells, whereas only 13 (14.1%) had CCR7 and 50 (54.3%) expressed CXCR4. The CXCR3, CXCR4, and CCR7 proteins were detected in the plasma membrane and cytoplasm of cancer cells. The normal epithelial cells of the colon did not express CXCR3, although some infiltrating inflammatory cells did. We then compared several clinicopathological factors between the cases with and without CXCR3 expression, and found a significant difference between the two groups in LN metastasis, TNM stage, lymphatic invasion, and vascular invasion. Regarding LN metastasis, 24 of 31 (77.4%) cases with CXCR3 expression metastasized to LNs, compared to 14 of 61 (22.9%) cases without CXCR3. On the other hand, there was no significant correlation between expression of CCR7 and these clinicopathological factors. Regarding CXCR4 expression, we found a significant difference between expression of CXCR4 and distant metastasis, vascular invasion, TNM stage, and LN metastasis. Among the 50 CXCR4-positive cases, 20 (80.0%) of 25 cases with CXCR3 metastasized to LNs, whereas only 6 (24.0%) of 25 cases without CXCR3 did ($P < 0.01$). We also determined independent risk factors for LN metastasis by a stepwise logistic regression analysis. According to the multivariate analysis of several variables, we found that CXCR3 expression and lymphatic invasion were significant independent risk factors. Finally, we examined the association of CXCR3 and/or CXCR4 expression with survival of the patients with colon cancers. Statistical analysis of the results by the log-rank (Mantel-Cox) test showed that the patients with CXCR3-positive tumors had a significantly poorer prognosis than those with CXCR3-negative tumors (Fig. 2D; $P < 0.01$). Importantly, the patients with CXCR4-positive tumors also had a significantly poorer prognosis, but its effect was less than CXCR3 (Fig. 2D; $P < 0.05$). In addition, the patients with tumors double positive for CXCR3 and CXCR4 had a significantly worse prognosis than those with tumors positive only for CXCR4 or double negative (Fig. 2D; $P < 0.01$). In contrast, expression of CCR7 had little effect on the patient survival. These results collectively indicate that expression of CXCR3 plays a pivotal role in LN metastasis of colon cancer and causes poorer prognosis.

Cancer Metastasis and Chemokine-Chemokine Receptor System

Metastasis is an inefficient process because it consists of multiple and complex steps, all of which must be successfully completed to give rise to the formation of metastatic tumors [12]. Recent studies suggest that the least-efficient steps in metastasis are the survival and growth of the micrometastatic foci and their persistence [2, 4], which indicates the importance of interactions between the "seed" (cancer cells) and "soil" (microenvironment). Accumulating evidence suggests that metastasis of tumors to specific organs can be aided by interactions between chemokine receptors on cancer cells and their ligands in the target organs. For example, CXCR4 stimulates metastasis of breast cancer and melanoma cells to the bone and lung where its ligand CXCL12 is abundant [24, 35]. It is also reported that metastasis of mouse colon cancer cell CT-26 to the liver and lung is greatly reduced if CXCR4 function is blocked [59]. Here, we have demonstrated that CXCR3 plays a critical role in LN metastasis of melanoma cells and colon cancer cells, without affecting that to the lung or liver [27, 28]. These results collectively suggest that distinct chemokine receptors control metastasis of tumor cells to specific organs; for example, CXCR3 to the lymph nodes and CXCR4 mainly to the lung and bone.

We have found that CXCL10 enhances the cell survival of melanoma and colon cancer cells in vitro, and that membranous expression of CXCR3 is upregulated upon serum starvation. It is therefore possible that membranous expression of CXCR3 is upregulated under various kinds of stress, which allows the tumor cells to survive and grow in a less-favorable microenvironment in distant organs. We have also demonstrated that DLD-1-CXCR3 cells disseminate to LNs at a similar frequency to that of DLD-1-EV cells 2 weeks after inoculation. By 4 weeks, however, more DLD-1-CXCR3 cells expanded rapidly than DLD-1-EV cells. It is conceivable that the presence of CXCR3 not only helps the initial dissemination of the cancer cells to the LNs, but also stimulates the growth and expansion of the metastatic foci in later stages by enhancing cell survival and gelatinase expression. On the other hand, B16F10 transfectants with reduced CXCR3 expression resulted in suppression of LN metastasis in both earlier and later stages [27], which suggests that it may depend on cell type how and when CXCR3 is involved in metastasis.

A complex network of chemokines and their receptors influences development of the primary tumors and their metastatic foci. The biological role of chemokines has two aspects in these processes: the role of chemokines in controlling leukocyte infiltration in cancer and the influence of chemokines on the metastatic potential and site-specific spread of tumor cells [1]. It has been demonstrated that CXCL9, CXCL10, and CCL21 exert antitumor activities by inducing immune-stimulating and angiostatic effects [49, 52]. Notably, CXCL9, CXCL10, and CCL21 play additional roles in the tumor microenvironment. For example, CXCL9 and CXCL10 activate RhoA and Rac1, induce actin reorganization, and trigger migration and invasion of melanoma, malignant B lymphocyte, and lung and breast cancers [45, 46, 50, 54]. We have demonstrated that CXCR3 plays a critical role in metastasis by inducing diverse cellular effects such as migration, invasion, and cell survival. Proinflammatory cytokines TNF-α and IFN-γ strongly stimulate the production of CXCL9, CXCL10, and CXCL11 in human intestinal epithelial cells [11]. Moreover, CXCL10 has been shown to be one of the Ras targets, and overexpressed in many cases of colorectal cancer [60]. It was also reported recently that CXCR3 expression was upregulated in metastatic colon cancer cells, but not in their primary counterparts, and that the CXCL10-CXCR3 axis significantly upregulated invasion-related properties in colon cancer [61]. The efficiency of chemotherapy may be improved significantly, if chemokine receptors are examined in biopsy and surgical samples, and a new strategy is added to inhibit the putative chemokine receptors responsible for metastasis.

Clinical Significance of LN Metastasis

Three viewpoints have been proposed on the basis of various hypotheses concerning the biology of distant metastasis development [43]. Throughout the first half of the twentieth century, the prevailing "Halstedian" theory, shaped by William Halsted, proposed that breast cancer begins as a strictly local disease and that tumor cells spread over time in a contiguous manner away from the primary site through lymphatics [17]. His idea provided justification for radical breast cancer surgery with lymphadenectomy. In the last half of the twentieth century, the "systemic" theory arose in reaction to the "Halstedian" theory. Bernard Fisher and others promulgated the view that breast cancer is a systemic disease at inception and that lymphadenectomy is merely useful for staging and does not affect overall survival [13]. Instead, the emphasis was on the importance of effective systemic therapy in breast cancer treatment, which has indeed been associated with substantial improvements of the overall survival. As a third hypothesis, the "spectrum" theory synthesized aspects of these two opposing approaches [18]. This view holds that there is a time when tumor cells have not metastasized to distant sites but that it is generally not known whether this time has passed at the point of diagnosis. According to this view, LN involvement is of prognostic importance not only because it indicates more malignant tumor biology, but also because persistent disease in LNs can be the source of subsequent fatal metastases. There is mounting evidence from prospective randomized clinical trials supporting a link between local control and overall survival in breast cancer. The Canadian and Danish trials demonstrated that the addition of radiation therapy after mastectomy and adjuvant chemotherapy not only decreased local recurrence, but also improved overall survival [41, 44]. A recent study by the Early Breast Cancer Trialists' Collaborative Group (EBCTCG) also presented the findings from 78 randomized clinical trials that improved local control at 5 years resulted in a highly statistically significant improvement in both breast cancer survival and overall survival at 15 years [5]. In addition to breast cancer, it was recently reported that extended LN dissection for gastric cancer has a significant long-term survival benefit over limited LN dissection by a prospective randomized trial [57]. These data imply that local disease is not only a marker of systemic disease but also a potential source for its future dissemination, and that local failure often leads to distant metastases that are likely eventually to decrease overall survival. Here, we have demonstrated that CXCR3 plays a critical role in LN metastasis of colon cancer, and that is associated with poorer prognosis. Taken together, CXCR3 can be a novel therapeutic target to suppress LN metastasis and to improve the overall survival in CXCR3-expressing cancers. Notably, systemic administration of a small molecular antagonist of CXCR3 (AMG487) has been recently reported to inhibit lung metastasis of breast cancer in a murine model, although the metastatic potential to LNs was not examined [54]. AMG487 is also currently being evaluated for efficacy in phase II clinical trials for psoriasis and rheumatoid arthritis [22].

Roles of Chemokine-Chemokine Receptor System in Other Aspects of Cancer Biology

In addition to metastasis, tumor promotion and growth are also aided by chemokines. Namely, CXCL14 helps recruitment of macrophages that promote hyperplastic tumors in the stomach [39]. In a breast cancer xenograft model, CXCL12 promotes angiogenesis by recruiting endothelial progenitor cells and stimulating tumor growth [38]. Our recent study has revealed an additional role of chemokines in tumor development, that is, promotion of tumor invasion by CCL9. These reports clearly indicate that chemokine-chemokine receptor interactions play important roles at various stages in tumor development.

In cancer tissues, the major source of chemokines including CXCL12 appears to be the stromal cells such as fibroblasts and leukocytes, although it remains unclear how genetic alterations in tumor cells cause the stromal cells to secrete chemokines. Our study has demonstrated that the tumor epithelial cells can secrete chemokine CCL9, through inactivation of the TGF-β family signaling. To our knowledge, this is the first demonstration that a genetic lesion, that is, loss of *Smad4* gene in the tumor epithelial cells can promote chemokine production that contributes to tumor invasion. Interestingly, another CC-chemokine CCL2 is produced by the tumor epithelium of human ovarian cancer and correlates with the extent of leukocyte infiltration and tumor progression [1]. These results suggest that recruitment of leukocytes by tumor cells themselves can promote tumor progression in various types of cancer, and that chemokines and their receptors may provide novel therapeutic targets.

In summary, chemokines are released locally and their effects are usually confined to local tissues, unlike cytokines that often cause systemic effects. Because of these characteristics, they can provide better targets for drug therapy that show less off-target side effects. Chemokine-chemokine receptor systems described in this chapter may provide examples of targets for anticancer therapeutics.

References

1. Balkwill, F. 2004. Cacner and the chemokine network. Nat. Rev. Cancer. 4:540–550.
2. Bao, S., Ouyang, G., Bai, X., Huang, Z., Ma, C., Liu, M., et al. 2004. Periostin potently promotes metastatic growth of colon cancer by augmenting cell survival via Akt/PKB pathway. Cancer Cell. 5:329–339.
3. Cella, M., Jarrossay, D., Facchetti, F., Alebardi, O., Nakajima, H., Lanzavecchia, A., et al. 1999. Plasmacytoid monocytes migrate to inflamed lymph nodes and produce large amounts of type I interferon. Nat. Med. 5:919–923.
4. Chambers, A. F., Groom, A. C., and MacDonald, I. C. 2002. Dissemination and growth of cancer cells in metastatic sites. Nat. Rev. Cancer. 2:563–572.
5. Clarke, M., Collins, R., Darby, S., et al. 2005. Effects of radiotherapy and of differences in the extent of surgery for early breast cancer on local recurrence and 15-year survival: an overview of the randomised trials. Lancet. 366:2087–2106.
6. Coussens, L. M., and Werb, Z. 2002. Inflammation and cancer. Nature. 420:860–867.
7. Coussens, L. M., Tinkle, C. L., Hanahan, D., and Werb, Z. 2000. MMP-9 supplied by bone marrow-derived cells contributes to skin carcinogenesis. Cell. 103:481–490.
8. Curino, A. C., Engelholm, L. H., Yamada, S. S., et al. 2005. Intracellular collagen degradation mediated by uPARAP/Endo180 is a major pathway of extracellular matrix turnover during malignancy. J. Cell Biol. 169:977–985.
9. Cyster, J. G. 1999. Chemokines and cell migration in secondary lymphoid organs. Science. 286:2098–2101.
10. Dijkstra, I. M., Hulshof, S., van der Valk, P., Boddeke, H. W., and Biber, K. 2004. Activity of human adult microglia in response to CC chemokine ligand 21. J. Immunol. 172:2744–2747.
11. Dwinell, M. B., Lugering, N., Eckmann, L., and Kagnoff, M. F. 2001. Regulated production of interferon-inducible T-cell chemoattractants by human intestinal epithelial cells. Gastroenterology. 120:49–59.
12. Fidler, I. J., and Kripke, M. L. 1977. Metastasis results from preexisting variant cells within a malignant tumor. Science. 197:893–895.
13. Fisher, B. 1980. Laboratory and clinical research in breast cancer – A personal adventure: The David A. Karnofsky Memorial Lecture. Cancer Res. 40:3863–3874.
14. Friedl, P., and Wolf, K. 2003. Tumor-cell invasion and migration: diversity and escape mechanisms. Nat. Rev. Cancer. 3:362–374.
15. Gao, J-L.,Wynn, T. A.,Chang, Y., et al. 1997. Impaired host defense, hematopoiesis, granulomatous inflammation and type 1-type 2 cytokine balance in mice lacking CC chemokine receptor 1. J. Exp. Med. 185:1959–1968.
16. Gocheva, V., and Joyce, J. A. 2007. Cysteine cathepsins and the cutting edge of cancer invasion. Cell Cycle. 6:60–64.
17. Halsted, W. S. 1907. The results of radical operations for the cure of carcinoma of the breast. Ann. Surg. 46:1–19.
18. Hellman, S. 1994. Karnofsky Memorial Lecture: natural history of small breast cancers. J. Clin. Oncol. 12:2229–2234.
19. Horuk, R. 2005. BX471: a CCR1 antagonist with anti-inflammatory activity in man. Mini. Rev. Med. Chem. 5:791–804.
20. Horuk, H., Clayberger, C., Krensky, A. M., et al. 2001. A non-peptide functional antagonist of the CCR1 chemokine receptor is effective in rat heart transplant rejection. J. Biol. Chem. 276:4199–4204.
21. Janatpour, M. J., Hudak, S., Sathe, M., Sedgwick, J. D., and McEvoy, L. M. 2001. Tumor necrosis factor-dependent segmental control of MIG expression by high endothelial venules in inflamed lymph nodes regulates monocyte recruitment. J. Exp. Med. 193:1375–1384.
22. Johnson, M., Li, A. R., Liu, J., et al. 2007. Discovery and optimization of a series of quinazolinone-derived antagonists of CXCR3. Bioorg. Med. Chem. Lett. 17:3339–3343.

23. Kalluri, R., and Zeisberg, M. 2006. Fibroblasts in cancer. Nat. Rev. Cancer. 6:392–401.
24. Kang, Y., Siegel, P. M., Shu, W., Drobnjak, M., Kakonen, S. M., Cordon-Cardo, C., et al. 2003. A multigenic program mediating breast cancer metastasis to bone. Cancer Cell. 3:537–549.
25. Karnoub, A. E., Dash, A. B., Vo, A. P., Sullivan, A., et al. 2007. Mesenchymal stem cells within tumour stroma promote breast cancer metastasis. Nature. 446:557–563.
26. Kashtan, H., Rabau, M., Mullen, J. B. M., Wong, A. H. C., Roder, J. C., Shpitz, B., et al. 1992. Intra-rectal injection of tumor cells: a novel animal model of rectal cancer. Surg. Oncol. 1:251–256.
27. Kawada, K., Sonoshita, M., Sakashita, H., et al. 2004. Pivotal role of CXCR3 in melanoma cell metastasis to lymph nodes. Cancer Res. 64:4010–4017.
28. Kawada, K., Hosogi, H., Sonoshita, M., et al. 2007. Chemokine receptor CXCR3 promotes colon cancer metastasis to lymph nodes. Oncogene. 26:4679–4688.
29. Kitamura, T., Kometani, K., Hashida, H., et al. 2007. SMAD4-deficient intestinal tumors recruit CCR1$^+$ myeloid cells that promote invasion. Nat. Genet. 39:467–475.
30. Kitamura, T., and Taketo, M. M. 2007. Keeping out bad guys: Gateway to the cellular target therapy. Cancer Res. 2007:1009–10102.
31. Liang, M., Mallari, C., Rosser, M., et al. 2000. Identification and characterization of a potent, selective, and orally active antagonist of the CC chemokine receptor-1. J. Biol. Chem. 275:19000–19008.
32. Lin, E. Y., Nguyen, A. V., Russel, R. G., and Pollard, J. W. 2001. Colony-stimulating factor 1 promotes progression of mammary tumors to malignancy. J. Exp. Med. 193:727–739.
33. Martin-Fontecha, A., Thomsen, L. L., Brett, S., Gerard, C., Lipp, M., Lanzavecchia, et al. 2004. Induced recruitment of NK cells to lymph nodes provides IFN-γ for T$_H$1 priming. Nat. Immunol. 5:1260–1265.
34. Mook, O. R. F., Frederiks, W. M., and Van Noorden, C. J. F. 2004. The role of gelatinases in colorectal cancer progression and metastasis. Biochim. Biopys. Acta. 1705:69–89.
35. Müller, A., Homey, B., Soto, H., Ge, N., Catron, D., Buchanan, M. E. et al. 2001. Involvement of chemokine receptors in breast cancer metastasis. Nature. 410:50–56.
36. Ninomiya, I., Terada, I., Yoshizumi, T., Takino, T., Nagai, N., Morita, A., et al. 2004. Anti-metastatic effect of capecitabine on human colon cancer xenografts in nude mouse rectum. Int. J. Cancer. 112:135–142.
37. Olumi, A. F., Grossfeld, G. D., Hayward, S. W., Carroll, P. R., Tlsty, T. D., and Cunha, G. R. 1999. Carcinoma-associated fibroblasts direct tumor progression of initiated human prostatic epithelium. Cancer Res. 59:5002–5011.
38. Orimo, A., Gupta, P. B., Sgroi, D. C., et al. 2005. Stromal fibroblasts present in invasive human breast carcinomas promote tumor growth and angiogenesis through elevated SDF-1/CXCL12 secretion. Cell. 121:335–348.
39. Oshima, H., Oshima, M., Inaba, K., and Taketo, M. M. 2004. Hyperplastic gastric tumors induced by activated macrophages in COX-2/mPGES-1 transgenic mice. EMBO. J. 23:1669–1678.
40. Overall, C. M., and Kleifeld, O. 2006. Validating matrix metalloproteinases as drug targets and anti-targets for cancer therapy. Nat. Rev. Cancer. 6:227–239.
41. Overgaard, M., Hansen, P. S., Overgaard, J., et al. 1997. Postoperative radiotherapy in high-risk premenopausal women with breast cancer who receive adjuvant chemotherapy. N. Engl. J. Med. 337:949–955.
42. Poggi, A., Carosio, R., Fenoglio, D., Brenci, S., Murdaca, G.,Setti, M., et al. 2004. Migration of Vδ1 and Vδ2 T cells in response to CXCR3 and CXCR4 ligands in healthy donors and HIV-1-infected patients: competition by HIV-1 Tat. Blood. 103:2205–2213.
43. Punglia, R. S., Morrow, M., Winer, E. P. and Harris, J. R. 2007. Local therapy and survival in breast cancer. N. Engl. J. Med. 356:2399–2405.
44. Ragaz, J., Jackson, S. M., Le, N., et al. 1997. Adjuvant radiotherapy and chemotherapy in node-positive premenopausal women with breast cancer. N. Engl. J. Med. 337:956–962.

45. Robledo, M. M., Barolomé, R. A., Longo, N., Rodríguez-Frade, J. M., Mellado, M., Longo, I., et al. 2001. Expression of functional chemokine receptors CXCR3 and CXCR4 on human melanoma cells. J. Biol. Chem. 276:45098–45105.
46. Soejima, K., and Rollins, B. J. 2001. A functional IFN-γ-inducible protein-10/CXCL10-specific receptor expressed by epthelial and endothelial cells that is neither CXCR3 nor clycosaminoglycan. J. Immunol. 167:6756–6582.
47. Soto, H., Wang, W., Strieter, R. M., Copeland, N. G., Gilbert, D. J., Jenkins, N. A. et al. 1998. The CC chemokine 6Ckine binds the CXC chemokine receptor CXCR3. Proc. Natl. Acad. Sci. USA. 95:8205–8210.
48. Takaku, K., Oshima, M., Miyoshi, H., Matsui, M., Seldin, M. F., and Taketo, M. M. 1998. Intestinal tumorigenesis in compound mutant mice of both *Dpc4* (*Smad4*) and *Apc* genes. Cell. 92:645–956.
49. Tannenbaum, C. S., Tubbs, R., Armstrong, D., Finke, J. H., Bukowski, R. M., and Hamilton, T. A. 1998. The CXC chemokine IP-10 and Mig are necessary for IL-12-mediated regression of the mouse RENCA tumor. J. Immunol. 161:927–932.
50. Trentin, L., Agostini, C., Facco, M., Piazza, F., Perin, A., Siviero, M., et al. 1999. The chemokine receptor CXCR3 is expressed on malignant B cells and mediates chemotaxis. J. Clin. Invest. 104:115–121.
51. Tsutsumi, S., Kuwano, H., Morinaga, N., Shimura, T., and Asao, T. 2001. Animal model of para-aortic lymph node metastasis. Cancer Lett. 169:77–85.
52. Vicari, A. P., Ait-Yahita, S., Chemin, K., Mueller, A., Zlotnick, A., and Caux, C. 2000. Antitumor effects of the mouse chemokine 6Ckine/SLC through angiostatic and immunological mechanism. J. Immunol. 165:1992–2000.
53. von Andrian, U. H., and Mempel, T. R. 2003. Homing and cellular traffic in lymph nodes. Nat. Rev. Immunol. 3:867–878.
54. Walser, T. C., Rifat, S., Ma, X., Kundu, N., Ward, C., Goloubeva, O., et al. 2006. Antagonism of CXCR3 inhibits lung metastasis in a murine model of metastatic breast cancer. Cancer Res. 66:7701–7707.
55. Wang, J. M., Deng, X., Gong, W., and Su, S. 1998. Chemokines and their role in tumor growth and metastasis. J. Immunol. Methods. 220:1–17.
56. Weinberg, R. A. 2007. Multi-step tumorigenesis. The biology of cancer (Garland Science) Ch. 11, 399–462.
57. Wu, C. W., Hsiung, C. A., Lo, S. S., et al. 2006. Nodal dissection for patients with gastric cancer: a randomised controlled trial. Lancet Oncol. 7:309–315.
58. Yoneyama, H., Narumi, S., Zhang, Y., Murai, M., Baggiolini, M., Lanzavecchia, A., et al. 2002. Pivotal role of dendritic cell-derived CXCL10 in the retention of T helper cell 1 lymphocytes in secondary lymph nodes. J. Exp. Med. 195:1257–1266.
59. Zeelenberg, I. S., Ruuls-Van Stalle, L., and Roos, E. 2003. The chemokine receptor CXCR4 is required for outgrowth of colon carcinoma micrometastasis. Cancer Res. 62:3833–3839.
60. Zhang, R., Zhang, H., Zhu, W., Pardee, A. B., Coffey, R. J. Jr., Liang, P., et al. 1997. Mob-1, a Ras target gene, is overexpressed in colorectal cancer. Oncogene. 14:1607–1610.
61. Zipin-Roitman, A., Meshel, T., Sagi-Assif, O., Shalmon, B., Avivi, C., et al. 2007. CXCL10 promotes invasion-related properties in human colorectal carcinoma cells. Cancer Res. 67:3396–3405.

The CXCR3/CXCL3 Axis in Cancer

Yanchun Li and Amy M. Fulton

Abstract CXCR3 is a G protein-coupled receptor that binds the chemokines CXCL9 (Mig), CXCL10 (IP-10), and CXCL11 (I-Tac). The murine receptor also binds CCL21. CXCR3 is expressed on activated T cells, B cells, Natural Killer (NK) cells, dendritic cells, mast cells, and endothelial cells, and has now been reported on many malignant cells. There are several CXCR3 variants: CXCR3-A promotes chemotaxis and also plays a role in cell survival, CXCR3-B activation leads to inhibited DNA synthesis and apoptosis but less is known regarding the pathophysiologic role of CXCR3-alt. Melanoma, breast, and colon cancer cell lines express CXCR3, however, expression levels are not correlated with metastatic potential. Nevertheless, gene silencing of CXCR3 reduces the number of lymph node metastases from implanted melanoma or colon cancers without affecting expansion of the primary tumor implant or dissemination to the lungs. Gene silencing or antagonism of CXCR3 with a small molecular weight (m.w.) antagonist also inhibits breast cancer metastasis but in this setting, pulmonary metastases are reduced by receptor blockade. In all three histologic types, CXCR3 expression is associated with a poorer prognosis. In clear cell renal carcinoma and in chronic lymphocytic leukemia the opposite correlation is observed, where low CXCR3 is associated with shorter survival. In spite of the demonstrated contribution of tumor-expressed CXCR3 in promoting tumor metastasis in several disease settings, local overexpression of CXCR3 ligands leads to tumor inhibition in several cancer models. Antiangiogenic properties of CXCR3 ligands as well as the ability to attract CXCR3+ T lymphocytes and NK cells to the tumor contribute to the protective mechanisms. Manipulation of the CXCR3/CXCL3 axis should be considered as a potential therapeutic approach to prevent cancer progression.

A.M. Fulton (✉)
Marlene and Stewart Greenebaum Cancer Center and Department of Pathology,
University of Maryland School of Medicine, Baltimore, MD 21201, USA
e-mail: afulton@umaryland.edu

A.M. Fulton (ed.), *Chemokine Receptors in Cancer*, Cancer Drug Discovery
and Development, DOI 10.1007/978-1-60327-267-4_5,
© Humana Press, a part of Springer Science+Business Media, LLC 2009

Properties of CXCR3

CXCR3, like many other chemokine receptors, mediates the migration of host cells to sites of inflammation or injury where ligands are highly expressed [1]. CXCR3 is a seven-transmembrane domain G-protein-coupled receptor; human and murine CXCR3 share 86% amino acid identity. CXCR3 is the common receptor for three ligands: CXCL9 (Mig), CXCL10 (IP-10), and CXCL11 (I-Tac) and, in the mouse, CCL21. CXCL9, 10, and 11 are induced by type I and II interferons and the receptor is expressed on many host cells including some subsets of activated T lymphocytes, B cells, NK cells, dendritic cells, and mast cells. Importantly, CXCR3 is expressed on endothelial cells and binding of cognate ligands has been shown to inhibit angiogenesis ([2] and see Chapter 8). CXCR3 activation is linked to several pathways including MAPK, Src, and PI3K signaling pathways [3, 4]. Several functional domains of CXCR3 have been identified. The membrane proximal carboxyl terminus of CXCR3 is critical to migration of T cells as well as ligand-induced receptor internalization and PKC activation but the third intracellular loop regulates integrin-dependent cellular adhesion and actin polymerization [4].

In addition to binding by multiple ligands, additional complexity is provided by the expression of several variants of CXCR3 in human cells. Lasagni et al. [5] first described an alternatively spliced variant of CXCR3, termed CXCR3-B. This mRNA resulted from initiation upstream of the known AG acceptor site and generated a 416-amino acid receptor with a longer NH2-terminal extracellular domain. The remainder of the protein was identical to the original CXCR3, now termed CXCR3-A. Transfection of CXCR3-A or CXCR3-B into a human microvascular endothelial cell line revealed different functions for these two receptors. CXCR3-A supported cell survival and chemotaxis by a pertussis-toxin sensitive mechanism. In contrast, CXCR3-B overexpression resulted in increased apoptosis and inhibition of DNA synthesis. Calcium mobilization by cells expressing CXCR3-A and induction of cAMP by CXCR3-B activation suggest that these variants are coupled to different intracellular signaling pathways. Evidence was provided that blood vessels associated with malignant tissues preferentially express CXCR-B indicating that the tumor neovasculature could be an attractive target for angiostatic actions of CXCR3 ligands.

A second CXCR3 variant has also been identified that is truncated at the C-terminus (CXCR3-alt, [6]). This altered receptor has a predicted four or five-transmembrane structure lacking the third and most of the second extracellular loop. In spite of the truncated form of CXCR3-alt, this variant was able to transduce a chemotactic signal by CXCL11 that was sensitive to inhibition by pertussis toxin.

CXCR3 plays a role in many other disorders. For example, CXCR3-positive T cells mediate several autoimmune disorders [7]. In the normal salivary gland, epithelial cells express CXCR3, which acts as a chemokine-scavenging receptor to control chemokine bioavailability. In the autoimmune disorder Sjogren's syndrome, the scavenging function of CXCR3 expressed on salivary gland epithelial cells is impaired. The authors suggest that the resulting greater bioavailability of circulating CXCR3 ligands could attract CXCR3+ T lymphocytes to the salivary gland driving further inflammation.

CXCR3 Expression in Malignancy

As described elsewhere in this volume, several chemokine receptors have been implicated in the behavior of various malignancies. The first studies to describe chemokine receptor expression in melanoma and breast cancer did not detect CXCR3 [8]; however, more recently, data in support of a role for CXCR3 has emerged in melanoma, neuroblastoma, and carcinoma of the colon, breast, ovary, prostate, kidney, and malignant B cells [9–16]. For many malignancies, CXCR3 expression is associated with more aggressive disease. Interestingly, in clear cell renal carcinoma and chronic lymphocytic leukemia the opposite relationship is observed; low CXCR3 expression is associated with a worse prognosis [17, 18]. Thus, the contribution of CXCR3 to tumor behavior cannot be generalized to all malignancies; however, a picture is emerging regarding the functional contribution of CXCR3 to malignancies of the breast, colon, and in melanoma.

Melanoma

Melanoma cell lines express CXCR3 and proliferation and migration are supported by the CXCR3 ligand, CXCL9 [14]. VLA-5- and VLA-4-dependent adhesion and activation of the small GTPases RhoA and Rac1 induce cytoskeletal rearrangements leading to cell migration. Ligand binding acti-vated the MAP kinases, p44/42 and p38, on melanoma cells. Kawada et al. first demonstrated a functional role for CXCR3 in mediating tumor metas-tasis ([12], also see Chapter 4). Using the B16 murine model of melanoma, the laboratory showed that CXCR3 expression levels do not differ in high-metastatic B16F10 versus low-metastatic B16F1 cells. Even though the expression levels do not correlate with clinical behavior, the functional importance of CXCR3 was demonstrated by studies showing that CXCR3-gene-silenced B16F10 melanoma cells developed fewer lymph node metastases than mice injected with control tumor cells. Unlike lymph node deposition, pulmonary metastases were not affected by altering levels of CXCR3. Likewise, growth of the primary tumors was not affected by the expression levels of CXCR3. Induction of an inflammatory response in the lymph nodes increased the local levels of CXCL9 and CXCL10, which directed more tumor cells to this site. This was the first study in vivo establishing a functional linkage between CXCR3 and tumor metastasis. These authors also examined the expression and function of CXCR3 ligands in melanoma. In contrast to some malignancies, melanoma cell lines do not endogenously express CXCR3 ligand mRNA. Addition of exogenous ligand to cultured melanoma cells also did not affect proliferation unless the cells were grown under serum-free conditions. In the latter condition, CXCL9 supported the survival of melanoma cells.

In a small series of biopsies, CXCR3 was detected in human melanoma but no correlation with clinical outcomes was examined [12]. More recently, others have examined CXCR3 expression by immunohistochemistry in a larger series of melanoma patients [19]. CXCR3 protein was detected in 32% of biopsies. CXCR3 expression was positively correlated with tumor thickness and the presence of distant metastases, lending further support to a role for CXCR3 in promoting melanoma metastasis to the lymph nodes.

Breast Cancer

Although it was initially reported that human breast cancer cell lines do not express CXCR3 [8], more recent studies show, by flow cytometry, that CXCR3 is widely expressed on breast cancer cell lines [9]. Receptor expression is increased in serum-starved cells. Unlike melanoma cells, malignant breast cells also express the CXCR3 ligand CXCL10 and, surprisingly, exposure of cells to exogenous ligand increases the detection of CXCR3.

Other laboratories have confirmed that human breast cancer cell lines express both CXCR3 and CXCL10 and the latter stimulates proliferation of these cells [20]. Dual expression of both ligand and receptor provides support for an autocrine loop whereby ligand supports the survival and growth of malignant breast cells. Ras activation further increased the expression of CXCL10. Evidence was also provided that both CXCR3-A and CXCR3-B are present on human breast cancer cell lines MDA-MB-435 and MCF-7. This study further confirmed the opposing role of these CXCR3 variants, originally described on endothelial cells, on malignant cell behavior. Gene silencing of CXCR3-B enhanced the ability of CXCL10 to support cell proliferation consistent with an inhibitory activity of CXCR3-B and indirectly providing evidence of a growth-promoting role for CXCR3-A. This CXCR3-B effect was not sensitive to inhibition by pertussis toxin and appears to confirm the initial study in microvascular endothelial cells that CXCR3-B is linked to inhibition of cell growth by a mechanism not coupled to Gi. Immunohistochemical examination of a small series of human breast cancer biopsies confirmed that both CXCR3 and CXCL10 are detected. The antibody to CXCR3 could not distinguish between CXCR3-A and CXCR3-B so the role of CXCR3 variants in primary breast cancers remains to be determined.

Our laboratory has also shown that murine and human breast cancer cell lines express CXCR3 mRNA and protein [21]. By flow cytometry, we observed that significantly more CXCR3 is detected in the cytoplasm than on the surface of tumor cells, an observation reported on other malignant and normal cells [22]. Receptor activation by CXCL9, CXCL10, or CXCL11 leads to calcium mobilization and a chemotactic response; however, CXCL10 and CXCL11 are more potent activators of these responses than CXCL9. Using a specific small m.w. antagonist of CXCR3, AMG487, we showed that lung-colonizing ability or spontaneous metastasis to the lungs from a mammary-gland-implanted tumor was inhibited by receptor antagonism. As reported in melanoma [12], we also did not observe any effect of CXCR3 antagonism on growth of the local breast tumor. These data are consistent with a trafficking role for CXCR3 whereby receptor-positive tumor cells migrate to the lungs, a demonstrated site of ligand expression. To determine if the host contributes to the therapeutic activity of receptor blockade, we compared the efficacy of AMG487 in immunologically intact as well as NK cell-depleted mice. When the host was depleted of NK cells, antimetastatic therapy of AMG487 was lost. We interpret these data to mean that interference with tumor cell trafficking is not sufficient to reduce metastasis; immune-mediated destruction of circulating tumor cells may also be necessary.

To confirm the central role of CXCR3 in breast tumor metastasis, we have recently derived mammary tumor cell lines that stably express shRNA targeting CXCR3 (Molecular Cancer Therapeutics 8:490, 2009). After transplantation of multiple gene-silenced tumor cell clones to syngeneic mice, we have observed that reduced CXCR3 is associated with markedly reduced pulmonary metastasis, consistent with our data using a pharmacologic CXCR3 antagonist. CXCR3 silencing does not affect the growth rate of the primary tumor. Thus, by two different approaches, we have shown that CXCR3, expressed on breast tumor cells contributes to the ability of these cells to metastasize to the lung but does not affect expansion of the primary tumor.

CXCR3 has been reported in human breast tumor biopsies [20], however, no information was available regarding the relationship of CXCR3 expression to clinical behavior. Using a tissue microarray comprised of 75 primary breast tumor specimens, we have now determined that CXCR3 is detected on the plasma membrane and in the cytoplasm of malignant epithelium from each patient. The degree of expression was correlated with overall and disease-free survival (Mol. Cancer Ther. 8:490, 2009); women with breast tumors expressing the highest levels of CXCR3 experienced the worst survival. Multivariant analysis established that CXCR3 was an independent predictor of a poor prognosis.

Colon Carcinoma

In addition to melanoma and breast cancer, colon carcinoma is the third malignancy in which CXCR3 has been most clearly implicated [13]. The Taketo laboratory had earlier shown that manipulation of CXCR3 in a murine model of melanoma determines successful dissemination to lymph nodes and this more recent study confirms the same relationship in colon cancer. Human colorectal carcinoma cells were engineered to express high levels of CXCR3 and implanted intrarectally into mice. The initial deposition in the lymph nodes was not different for high versus low CXCR3-expressing cells, however expansion of tumors into macroscopic colonies was accelerated by high CXCR3. In contrast, dissemination to the lungs or liver was not affected by changes in CXCR3 expression levels. As observed in melanoma and breast cancer, inhibition of CXCR3 function in colon cancer does not affect the growth pattern of the primary tumor.

The addition of CXCL10 to cultured cells supported increased cell survival, but this effect was only observed in serum-free culture conditions. Ligand stimulation resulted in calcium mobilization, ERK1/2 and AKT phosphorylation, and the induction of MMP2 and MMP9. These investigators also demonstrated that CCL21 acted as a ligand for CXCR3 since cellular responses were inhibited with antibody to CXCR3. Low-serum conditions also increased the detection of surface CXCR3. The expression of CXCR3 was examined in biopsy material. By immunohistochemistry, 34% of the samples examined had detectable CXCR3; CXCR3-positive tumors were more likely to come from patients with nodal involvement and, importantly, CXCR3 expression was associated with poorer overall survival.

All known variants of CXCR3 (CXCR3-A, CXCR3-B, and CXCR3-alt) were detected on colon cancer cell lines [23]. CXCL10 induced migration, adhesion, and MMP9 secretion. CXCR3 was also detected in colon cancer biopsies (the antibody could not distinguish CXCR3 variants). Thus, there is considerable support for the important role of CXCR3 in colon cancer.

Prostate Cancer

Like breast cancer, prostate cancer cell lines express both CXCR3 and CXCR3 ligands at both the mRNA and protein levels [15]. Expression of both ligand and receptor has been confirmed in prostate cancer cells in two other laboratories [24, 25]. Forced overexpression of CXCL10 resulted in lower proliferation rates and decreased PSA production. Also, as reported for breast cancer cells, increased ligand expression led to upregulation of receptor. Shen et al. used the transgenic TRAMP model of prostate cancer to investigate the role of host CXCR3 in tumor behavior [24]. When TRAMP mice were crossed with CXCR3-/- mice, spontaneous prostate tumors appeared earlier and expanded more rapidly in comparison to TRAMP tumors in CXCR3 +/+ mice. These authors conclude that the more aggressive behavior of prostate cancers in the absence of host CXCR3 expression is attributable to the loss of CXCR3 on endothelial cells. Binding of CXCR3 ligands to endothelium inhibits proliferation of blood vessels. It is also possible that the absence of host immune cells, notably, CXCR3+ T lymphocytes and NK cells, contributes to more aggressive prostate cancer in this setting.

Other Solid Tumors

CXCR3 expression has also been observed in other malignancies including ovarian carcinoma and in neuroblastoma cell lines [10, 26]. During progression from endometriosis to frank ovarian tumors, host CXCR3 expression wanes, whereas receptor expression is increased in malignant epithelium [26]. Concurrently, CXCL11 levels increased. The authors suggest that the beneficial effects of CXCL11 on host T-cell activation are lost during tumor progression and that ultimately, CXCL11 supports tumor cell growth.

Exceptions to the Rule

We have summarized many reports indicating that tumor CXCR3 contributes to tumor progression. There are several interesting exceptions to this observation. A recent paper describes CXCR3 expression in 96% of clear cell renal cell carcinoma specimens examined [17]. Low expression, rather than high expression, is associated with a worse prognosis. Five-year disease-free survival was observed in 57% of patients with low-CXCR3 tumors, but 82% of patients with high-CXCR3 tumors were alive at 5 years. In multivariant analysis, CXCR3 was shown to be an independent prognostic factor. The authors posit that the anti-angiogenic effects of CXCR3 and/or host CXCR3+ cells are protective. These studies indicate that it will be important to delineate the distinct roles of CXCR3 expressed on malignant versus host cells. CXCR3 has also been described on malignant B cells [11, 16]. CXCR3 was detected on specimens from all 31 patients with chronic lymphocytic leukemia [16], but not on B cells from healthy individuals. Malignant, CXCR3-positive cells migrated in vitro in response to stimulation with CXCL9 or CXCL10. Although these studies were consistent with a promalignancy role for CXCR3, a recent study reached the opposite conclusion. Low CXCR3 expression was associated with a poor prognosis in CLL [18].

As reported in RCC, low CXCR3 was an independent predictor of shorter survival, by multivariant analysis.

What Are the Roles of CXCR3 Ligands in Tumor Behavior?

CXCR3 ligands have been detected in several tumors. Higher expression is generally associated with less-aggressive disease, increased T-cell infiltrate, and decreased microvessel density [27, 28]. In renal cell carcinoma, mRNA for CXCL9 and CXCL10 were detected at higher levels in malignant versus normal tissue. A positive correlation was observed between levels of ligands and absence of tumor recurrence [27]. In melanoma, a positive association was observed between the degree of T-cell infiltration and levels of CXCR3 ligands, suggesting that ligand attracted CXCR3+ T cells to the tumor site [28]. CXCL11 mRNA was detected in human breast cancers and surrounding normal tissue. Message levels were higher in stage I or II disease versus more advanced disease [29]. Addition of recombinant CXCL9, CXCL10, or CXCL11 has variously been shown to inhibit, stimulate, or have no effect on proliferation of tumor cell lines. In most examples, the effects of ligand on tumor cell proliferation are modest. This is a complex question since ligand can affect tumor cell behavior not only through actions on CXCR3 expressed on the malignant cell, but also on the many other cells (endothelial, Th1 T lymphocytes, cytotoxic CD8+ T cells, activated B cells, and NK cells) that express CXCR3. In particular, endogenous CXCR3 ligands are central to the development of effective antitumor cytotoxic effector cells. Activated CD4+ and CD8+ T lymphocytes and NK cells express CXCR3 and each effector population can contribute to tumor control.

An intriguing recent study shows that advanced cutaneous T-cell lymphoma is associated with downregulation of surface expression of CXCR3 on normal CD8+ T cells in the circulation of patients [30]. CXCR3 transcript levels were normal or elevated in patients; however, CXCR3 protein was sequestered in the cytoplasm. The cytotoxic activity of these CD8+ cells was preserved but the capacity to migrate in response to CXCR3 ligands was reduced in comparison to CD8+ cells from healthy donors. Circulating ligand was also detected during disease progression. These findings support the hypothesis that circulating ligands lead to downregulation of CXCR3 on CD8+ cytotoxic T cells compromising the ability of these effector cells to migrate into malignant cutaneous lesions. Thus, a novel mechanism of immune suppression could be mediated by excess production of CXCR3 ligands. As described earlier, in the autoimmune disease Sjogren's syndrome, it has been proposed that epithelial cells expressing CXCR3 can scavenge CXCR3 ligands, rendering them unavailable to direct the migration of effector T and/or NK cells [7]. Tumor CXCR3 could play a similar role in ovarian carcinoma [26]. In primary lymphoma, EBV-encoded microRNA (miRNA) was expressed endogenously and was inversely correlated with levels of CXCL11 suggesting that EBV miRNA suppresses CXCL11 expression [31]. Lower CXCL11 would be predicted to suppress the localization of effector T cells. If confirmed, this finding represents a novel mechanism by which tumor could suppress effective antitumor T-cell responses.

In contrast to the tumor growth-promoting qualities of endogenous ligands, there are numerous examples in which overexpressed CXCL9, CXCL10, or CXCL11 leads to tumor inhibition in cancer models of breast, renal cell, lung, neuroblastoma [32–38]. One of the earliest studies describing antitumor activity of IP-10 showed that this protective effect was dependent on host T cells [33]. Direct intratumor injection of recombinant CXCL9 or CXCL10 limits growth of Burkitts lymphoma [34]. We have engineered murine mammary tumor cells to overexpress CXCL9 and shown that chemokine-mediated inhibition of tumors growing in the mammary gland is dependent on CD4+ and CD8+ T lymphocytes [37, 38]. CXCL9-expressing tumors also contain more CD4+CXCR3+ as well as CD8+CXCR3+ T cells than tumors expressing the control vector. Increased numbers of CD4+, interferon-γ-positive T cells were also observed in Mig-expressing tumors.

While there is general agreement that high expression of CXCL9, CXCL10, or CXCL11 can suppress tumor growth in many models, the mechanisms of inhibition differ. Our studies and others have confirmed a critical role of T lymphocytes in the mechanism by which Mig, IP-10, and I-Tac suppress tumor growth in some models [33, 38]. Other studies demonstrate that CXCR3 ligands can mediate tumor inhibition even in T-cell deficient mice indicating that other T-cell independent mechanisms are also important. For example, many labs have shown that angiostatic properties of CXCR3 ligands contribute to tumor control [2, 34–36]. Elsewhere in this volume, Streiter and co-authors describe studies, which identified the angiostatic activity of ELR-negative chemokines including CXCL9-11. The angiostatic activities of these ligands are mediated through the CXCR3-B receptor expressed on endothelial cells.

While many studies have examined the ability of CXCR3 ligands to control local tumor growth, using a model of metastatic breast cancer, we have also demonstrated that CXCL9 is effective at controlling tumor metastasis [38]. In this setting, NK cells, rather than T lymphocytes, play a critical role in the therapeutic response. Thus, both T cells and NK cells may be targeted therapeutically by enhancing the intratumor levels of CXCR3 ligands. High circulating levels of CXCL9 alone are not sufficient to induce a protective response in a murine model of renal cell carcinoma [36]. Presumably this is because a chemokine gradient is not produced which would direct protective host cells to the tumor. An effective chemokine gradient was necessary in which the ligand was expressed directly in the tumor site and this approach was combined with systemic IL-2 to induce expression of CXCR3 on the host cells. We have also proposed that by inducing higher chemokine concentrations in the tumor we are effectively reversing the chemokine gradient resulting in diminished migration of the tumor cells out of the primary tumor (Fig. 1).

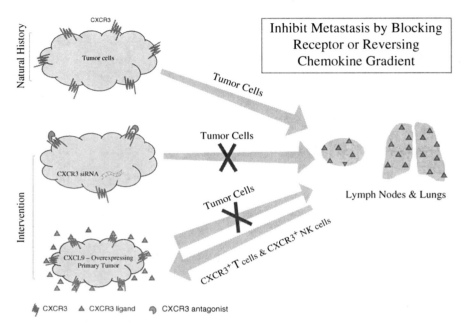

Fig. 1 Breast and other malignant epithelial cells constitutively express CXCR3 but little or no CXCR3 ligand is expressed in the primary tumor site. CXCR3-positive tumor cells migrate in response to the chemokine gradient to sites where CXCR3 ligands are expressed (lymph nodes, lung). Therapeutic interventions to reduce tumor-CXCR3 signaling include gene silencing of CXCR3 or small m.w. receptor antagonists. By blocking tumor-CXCR3, metastasis in response to the chemokine gradient is inhibited. Alternatively, forced intratumoral expression of CXCR3 ligands, in this example, CXCL9, reduces metastatic potential by reversing the chemokine gradient and attracting CXCR3+ T cells and NK cells to the primary tumor site

Summary

Several laboratories have provided evidence that expression of CXCR3 on malignant cells supports tumor metastasis. Several genetic and pharmacologic approaches have identified possible strategies to block CXCR3 signaling. Paradoxically, overexpression of CXCR3 ligands is therapeutic in many tumor models. This clearly is a function, in part, of the different effects of ligand binding on different CXCR3-positive cells. Furuya has shown that in benign ovarian disease, CXCR3 is chiefly detected on host cells, but CXCR3-positive lymphocytes decrease in proportion to CXCR3-positive tumor cells in ovarian carcinoma [26]. Although it might be predicted that systemic antagonism of CXCR3 would be detrimental to host immune effector cell function, thus promoting tumor growth, our initial studies with systemic receptor blockade have not supported this hypothesis ([21] and unpublished data). We have observed no effect of systemic CXCR3 inhibition on local tumor growth even in the presence of potent antimetastatic activity. The opposite approach of intentional overexpression of CXCR3 ligands also has demonstrated antitumor activity in many model systems. It may be challenging to extrapolate these latter findings to the clinical setting. Different levels of ligand expression and different sites of expression (systemic versus local) may have contrasting roles in tumor behavior because they act on different CXCR3-positive populations. Nevertheless, the data are compelling that CXCR3, expressed on some, but not all, malignant cells, contributes to metastatic capacity. CXCR3 should be considered as a potential therapeutic target to inhibit tumor metastasis.

References

1. Lazzeri E, Romagnani P. CXCR3-binding chemokines: novel multifunctional therapeutic targets. Curr. Drug Targets Immunol. Endocr Metabol Disord. 5:109–18, 2005.
2. Arenberg DA, Kunkel SL, Polverini PJ, Morris SB, Burdick MD, Glass MC, Taub DT, Iannettoni MD, Whyte RI, Streiter RM. Interferon-γ-inducible protein 10 (IP-10) is an angiostatic factor that inhibits human non-small cell lung cancer (NSCLC) tumorigenesis and spontaneous metastases. J. Exp. Med. 184:981–992, 1996.
3. Shahabuddin S, Ji R, Wang P, Brailoiu E, Dun N, Yang Y, Aksoy MO, Kelsen SG. CXCR3 chemokine receptor-induced chemotaxis in human airway epithelial cells: role of p38 MAPK and PI3K signaling pathways. Am. J. Cell Physiol. 291:C34–9, 2006.
4. Dagan-Berger M, Feniger-Barish, Avniel S, Wald H, Galun E, Brabovsky V, Alon R, Nagler A, Ben-Baruch A, Peled A. Role of CXCR3 carboxyl terminus and third intracellular loop in receptor-mediated migration, adhesion and internalization in response to CXCL11. Blood 107:3821–31, 2006.
5. Lasagni L, Francalanci M, Annunziato F, Lazzeri E, Giannini S, Cosmi L, Sagrinati C, Mazzinghi B, Orlando C, Maggi E, Marra F, Romagnani S, Serio M, Romagnani, P. An alternatively spliced variant of CXCR3 mediates the inhibition of endothelial cell growth induced by IP-10, Mig and I-TAC and acts as functional receptor for platelet factor 4. J. Exp. Med. 197:1537–1549, 2003.
6. Ehlert JE, Addison CA, Burdick MD, Kunkel SL, Strieter, RM. Identification and partial characterization of a variant of human CXCR3 generated by posttranscriptional exon skipping. J. Immunol. 173:6234–6240, 2004.
7. Sfriso P, Oliviero F, Calabrese F, Miiorin M, Faco M, Contri A, Cabrelle A, Baesso I, Cozzi F, Andretta M, Cassatella MA, Fiocco U, Todesco S, Konttinen YT, Punzi L, Agostini C. Epithelial CXCR3-B regulates chemokines bioavailability in normal, but not in Sjogren's syndrome salivary glands. J. Immunol. 176:2581–2589, 2006.
8. Muller A, Homey B, Soto H, Ge N, Catron D, Buchanan ME, McClanahan T, Murphy E, Yuan W, Wagner SN, Barrera JL, Mohar A Verastegui E, Zlotnik A. Involvement of chemokine receptors in breast cancer metastasis. Nature 410:50–6, 2001.
9. Goldberg-Bittman L, Neumark E, Sagi-Assif O, Azenshtein E, Meshel T, Witz IP, Ben-Baruch, A. The expression of the chemokine receptor CXCR3 and its ligand, CXCL10, in human breast adenocarcinoma cell lines. Immunol. Lett. 92:171–8, 2004.
10. Goldberg-Bittman L, Sagi-Assif O, Meshel T, Nevo I, Levy-Nissenbaum O, Yron I, Witz IP, Ben-Baruch A. Cellular characteristics of neuroblastoma cells: Regulation by the ELR⁻- CXC chemokine CXCL10 and expression of a CXCR3-like receptor. Cytokine 29:105–17, 2005.

11. Jones D, Benjamin RJ, Shahsafaei A, Dorfman DM. The chemokine receptor CXCR3 is expressed in a subset of B-cell lymphomas and is a marker of B-cell chronic lymphocytic leukemia. Blood 95:627–32, 2000.
12. Kawada K, Sonoshita M, Sakashita H, Takabayashi A, Yamaoka Y, Manabe T, Inaba K, Minato N, Oshima M, Taketo MM. Pivotal role of CXCR3 in melanoma cell metastasis to lymph nodes. Cancer Res. 64:4010–7, 2004.
13. Kawada K, Hosogi H, SonoshitaM, Sakashita H, Manabe T, Shimahara Y, Sakai Y, Takabayashi A, Oshima M, Taketo MM. Chemokine receptor CXCR3 promotes colon cancer metastasis to lymph nodes. Oncogene 26:4679–4688, 2007.
14. Robledo MM, Bartolome RA, Longo N, Rodriguez-Frade JM, Mellado M, Longo I, van Muijen GN, Sanchez-Mateos, Teixido J. Expression of functional chemokine receptors CXCR3 and CXCR4 on human melanoma cells. J. Biol. Chem. 276: 45098–105, 2001.
15. Engl T, Relja B, Blumenberg C, et al. Prostate tumor CXC-chemokine profile correlates with cell adhesion to endothelium and extracellular matrix. Life Sci. 78:1784–93, 2006.
16. Trentin L, Agostini C, Facco M, Piazza F, Perin A, Siviero M, Gurrieri C, Galvan S, Adami F, Zambello R, Semenzato G. The chemokine receptor CXCR3 is expressed on malignant B cells and mediates chemotaxis. J. Clin. Invest. 104:115–21, 1999.
17. Klatte T, Seligson DB, Leppert JT, Riggs SB, Yu H, Zomorodian N, Kabbinavar FF, Strieter RM, Belldegrun AS, Pantuck AJ. The chemokine receptor CXCR3 is an independent prognostic factor in patients with localized clear cell renal cell carcinoma. J. Urol. 179:61–66, 2008.
18. Ocana E, Delgado-Perez L, Campos-Caro A, Munoz J, Paz A, Franco R, Brieva JA. The prognostic role of CXCR3 expression by chronic lymphocytic leukemia B cells. Haematologica 92:349–356, 2007.
19. Monteagudo C, Martin JM, Jorda E, Llombart-Bosch A. CXCR3 chemokine receptor immunoreactivity in primary cutaneous malignant melanoma:correlation with clinicopathologic prognostic factors. J. Clin. Pathol. 60:596–9, 2007.
20. Datta D, Flaxenburg JA, Laxmanan S, Geehan C, Grimm M, Waaga-Gasser AM, Briscoe DM, and Pal S. Ras-induced modulation of CXCL10 and its receptor splice variant CXCR3-B in MDA-MB-435 and MCF-7 cells: relevance for the development of human breast cancer. Cancer Res. 66:9509–9518, 2006.
21. Walser TC, Rifat S, Ma X, Kundu N, Ward C, Goloubeva O, Johnson MG, Medina JC, Collins TL, Fulton AM. Antagonism of CXCR3 inhibits lung metastasis in a murine model of metastatic breast cancer. Cancer Res. 66:7701–7707, 2006.
22. Aksoy MO, Yang Y, Ji R, Reddy PJ, Shahabuddin S, Litvin J, Rogers TJ, Kelsen SG. CXCR3 surface expression in human airway epithelial cells:cell cycle dependence and effect on cell proliferation. Am. J. Physiol. Lung Cell Mol. Physiol. 290:L909–18, 2005.
23. Zipin-Roitman A, Meshel T, Sagi-Assif O, Shalmon B, Avivi C, Pfeffer RM, Witz IP, Ben-Baruch A. CXCL10 promotes invasion-related properties in human colorectal carcinoma cells. Cancer Res. 67:3396–3405, 2007.
24. Shen H, Schuster R, Lu B, Waltz SE, Lentsch AB. Critical and opposing roles of the chemokine receptors CXCR2 and CXCR3 in prostate tumor growth. Prostate 66: 1721–1728, 2006.
25. Nagpal ML, Davis J, Lin T. Overexpression of CXCL10 in human prostate LnCaP cells activates its receptor (CXCR3) expression and inhibits cell proliferation. Biochim. Biophys. Acta 1762:811–818, 2006.
26. Furuya M, Suyama T, Usui H, Kasuya Y, Nishiyama M, Tanaka N. et al. Up-regulation of CXC chemokines and their receptors: implications for proinflammatory microenvironments of ovarian carcinomas and endometriosis. Human Path. 38: 1676–1687, 2007.
27. Kondo T, Ito F, Nakazawa H, Horita S, Osaka Y and Toma H. High expression of chemokine gene as a favorable prognostic factor in renal cell carcinoma. J. Urol. 171: 2171–5, 2004.

28. Kunz M, Toksoy A, Goebeler M, Engelhardt E, Brocker E, Gillitzer R. Strong expression of the lymphoattractant CXC chemokine Mig is associated with heavy infiltration of T cells in human malignant melanoma. J. Pathol. 189: 52–8, 1999.

29. Chu Y, Yang X, Xu W, Wang Y., Guo Q., Xiong S. In situ expression of IFN-γ-inducible T cell α chemoattractant in breast cancer mounts an enhanced specific anti-tumor immunity which leads to tumor regression. Cancer Immunol. Immunother. 56: 1539–1549, 2007.

30. Winter D, Moser J, Kriehuber E, Wiesner C, Knobler R, Trautinger F, Bombosi P, Stingl, G, Petzelbauer P, Rot A, Maurer D. Down modulation of CXCR3 surface expression and function in CD8+ T cells from cutaneous T cell lymphoma patients. J. Immunol. 179: 4272–82, 2007.

31. Xia T, O'Hara A, Araujo I, Barreto J, Carvalho E, Sapucaia JB, Ramos JC, Luz E, Pedroso C, Manrique M, Toomey NL, Brites C, Dittmer DP, Harrington, WJ. EBV microRNAs in primary lymphomas and targeting of CXCL-11 by ebv-mir-BHRF1-3. Cancer Res. 68: 1436–1442, 2008.

32. Tominaga M, Isashita Y, Ohta M, Shibata K, Ishio T, Ohmori N, Goto T, Sato S, Kitano S. Antitumor effects of the MIG and IP-10 genes transferred with poly [D,L-2,4-diaminobutyric acid] on murine neuroblastoma. Cancer Gene Ther. 14:696–705, 2007.

33. Luster AD, Leder P. IP-10, a CXC chemokine, elicits a potent thymus-dependent anti-tumor response in vivo. J. Exp. Med. 178:1057–1065, 1993.

34. Sgadari C, Angiolillo AL, Cherney BW, Pike SE, Farber JM, Koniaris LG, Vanguri P, Burd PR, Sheikh N, Gupta G, Teruya-Feldstein J, Tosato G. Interferon-inducible protein-10 identified as a mediator of tumor necrosis in vivo. Proc. Natl. Acad Sci. 93: 13791–13796, 1996.

35. Feldman AL, Friedl J, Lans TE, Libutti SK, Lorang D, Miller MS, Turner EM, Hewitt SM, Alexander HR. Retroviral gene transfer of interferon-inducible protein 10 inhibits growth of human melanoma xenografts. Int. J. Cancer 99:149–153, 2002.

36. Pan J, Burdick MD, Belperio JA, Xue YY, Gerard C, Sharma S, Dubinett SM, and Strieter RM. CXCR3/CXCR3 ligand biological axis impairs RENCA tumor growth by a mechanism of immunoangiostasis. J. Immunol. 176:1456–1464, 2006.

37. Dorsey R, Kundu N, Yang Q, Tannenbaum CS, Sun H, Hamilton TA, Fulton AM. Immunotherapy with interleukin-10 depends on the CXC chemokines inducible Protein-10 and Monokine induced by IFN-γ. Cancer Res. 62: 2606–2610, 2002.

38. Walser TC, Ma X, Kundu N, Dorsey R, Goloubeva O, Fulton AM. Immune-mediated modulation of breast cancer growth and metastasis by the chemokine Mig (CXCL9) in a murine model. J. Immunother. 30:490–498, 2007.

Roles for CCR7 in Cancer Biology

Lei Fang and Sam T. Hwang

Abstract Since 2001, the association of CCR7 expression by tumor cells with LN metastasis (and associated poor clinical outcome) has been validated in a large number of solid tumors as well as in hematopoietic malignancies. Local factors such as hypoxia, cytokines (endothelins), or epigenetic changes may be involved in the upregulation of CCR7 by tumor cells. Through distinct signaling pathways, activation of CCR7 by its cognate ligands, CCL21 or CCL19, promotes migration, invasion and proliferation of tumor cells *in vitro*. In addition to responding to exogenous sources of CCR7 ligands, CCR7-expressing tumor cells facilitate their own migration towards CCL21-expressing lymphatics by generating transcellular gradients of CCL19/21. While CCR7 antagonists appear to block LN metastasis in short-term experimental models, the dual roles of CCR7 in protective immunity and tolerance suggests that these agents must be carefully evaluated. Meanwhile, increasing CCR7 expression in DCs may represent a potentially useful means of improving the efficacy of *in vivo* DC vaccination strategies.

Introduction

Nearly all of the chemokine receptors involved in cancer progression, tumorigenesis, and metastasis have key functions in normal tissue homeostasis, trafficking, and survival. The subject of this chapter, CC chemokine receptor 7 (CCR7), is no exception. Under physiologic conditions, CCR7 and its two ligands play important roles in controlling the trafficking of a variety of leukocytes (several subsets of T cells and dendritic cells (DCs)) to secondary lymphoid organs such as the peripheral lymph nodes (LN). While early studies suggested that CCR7 regulated both chemotaxis and integrin-mediated

S.T. Hwang (✉)
Department of Dermatology, Medical College of Wisconsin, Milwaukee, WI 53226, USA
e-mail: sthwang@mcw.edu

A.M. Fulton (ed.), *Chemokine Receptors in Cancer*, Cancer Drug Discovery and Development, DOI 10.1007/978-1-60327-267-4_6,
© Humana Press, a part of Springer Science+Business Media, LLC 2009

adhesion step of leukocytes to vascular endothelium, recent studies suggest that CCR7 controls the cytoarchitecture, speed of migration, and maturation of leukocytes as well [1]. Given the known function of CCR7 in LN trafficking, it is not surprising that expression of CCR7 by cancer cells in experimental models leads to enhanced LN metastasis. In clinical studies, expression of CCR7 has been linked with a greater incidence of tumor LN metastases, which in human cancer patients is nearly always associated with poor outcomes. This review will focus on the expression patterns and functions of CCR7 and its ligands in normal physiology and in cancer biology.

Expression of CCR7 and Its Ligands

The two major leukocyte subsets that express CCR7 are DCs and T cells. While little or no CCR7 is present in resting, unactivated DCs, it becomes highly expressed in DCs upon tissue injury or with activation by cytokines such as TNF-α [2]. Naïve and central memory T cells constitutively express CCR7 as a means to recirculate continuously through secondary LN [3]. CCR7 is also expressed by $CD4^+CD25^+$ T regulatory cells that express FoxP3; indeed, CCR7-deficient T regulatory cells fail to suppress antigen-induced T-cell responses [4], suggesting that CCR7 is involved in the maintenance of tolerance as well as protective immunity [5].

CCL21 and CCL19 are the two physiologic ligands for CCR7 [6]. CCL21, also called secondary lymphoid tissue chemokine (SLC) or 6Ckine, is constitutively expressed on high endothelial venules (HEVs) of LNs and Peyer's patches, on lymphatic endothelium of multiple organs, and by stromal cells in T-cell areas of LNs, spleen, and Peyer's patches [7–9]. CCL19, also named ELC or MIP-3β, is expressed by stromal cells in T-cell areas of secondary lymphoid organs [10–12].

Naïve T cells and central memory T cells [13] continuously circulate through secondary lymphoid organs, where they may meet antigen-presenting cells (e.g., DCs) that carry cognate antigens. These T-cell subsets roll and tether along specialized vessels called HEVs in a selectin-dependent manner. Moreover, the interactions between CCL21 and CCR7 induce integrin-mediated firm adhesion of circulating lymphocytes to the endothelium of HEVs, leading to rapid transendothelial migration [14]. After encountering antigens in the periphery, immature DCs capture, process, and present antigens on their surface and differentiate into mature DCs that upregulate MHC II, costimulatory molecules, as well as CCR7. CCR7 and CCL21 are crucial for trafficking of mature DCs through afferent lymphatics into LNs [2, 3, 9]. Upon entering LNs, naïve T cells and mature DCs migrate in response to chemotactic gradients of CCL19 and CCL21 that are expressed by stromal cells within T-cell zones. In the T-cell zones, interactions between DCs and T cells foster both positive and inhibitory signals to the adaptive immune system [3, 5].

The importance of CCL21/CCL19 and CCR7 in T cell and DC homing to secondary lymphoid organs is supported by the observations from CCR7-deficient mice as well as from homozygous plt (paucity of lymph node T cells) mice, which have spontaneous mutations in CCL21 and CCL19 genes in secondary lymphoid organs [3, 15]. Plt mice were deficient in T cell and DC trafficking into regional LNs, more susceptible to infection, and unable to mount primary immune responses.

Interestingly, CCR7-deficient mice (compared to wild-type (WT) mice) showed augmented immune responses when repeatedly challenged with topical contact sensitizers. Moreover, CD4$^+$FoxP3$^+$ regulatory T cells were consistently reduced in peripheral LN, but not in spleen or blood, of CCR7-deficient (vs. WT) mice [4]. Finally, adoptively transferred CCR7-deficient T regulatory cells were not able to suppress antigen-induced T-cell responses present in an experimental inflammatory bowel disease [4]. By contrast, Krautwald and colleagues reported that CCL19-Ig impaired immune cell trafficking and blocked allograft rejection [16]. Moreover, they observed that, at high concentrations, CCL19 and CCL21 signaling inhibited T-cell proliferation [17]. These data suggest that CCR7 is crucial for the trafficking of regulatory (as well as effector) T cells to LN.

CCR7 in Cancer Biology

Cancer metastases share many similarities with leukocyte trafficking. Chemokine receptors such as CCR7, CXCR4, and CCR10 are often found upregulated in many types of human cancers and have been shown to play nonredundant roles in metastases by regulating cancer cell trafficking and survival [18, 19]. LNs are one of the common sites for cancer metastasis and nodal metastasis is highly associated with poor prognosis in many cancers. In this chapter, we will focus on the effects of CCR7 upregulation by cancer cells on LN metastasis and other pathological and clinical features, the underlying mechanisms that promote nodal metastasis and CCR7 upregulation by cancer cells, and the effects of CCR7 expression by CD8 T cells and mature DCs in cancer immunotherapy.

CCR7 Expression by Human Cancers and Its Correlation with Nodal Metastases and Poor Prognosis

In 2001, Mueller et al. first reported that several chemokine receptors, including CCR7, were upregulated on breast cancers and malignant melanoma in a distinct and nonrandom pattern [18]. They investigated the expression of chemokine receptors in breast cancer cell lines and malignant melanoma cell lines compared to normal primary mammary epithelial cells and normal primary melanocytes, respectively, using quantitative real-time PCR. CCR7 was consistently upregulated in both breast cancer and melanoma cell lines, a finding they confirmed in primary breast tumors. In addition, the most abundant expression of CCL21 mRNA was found in human LNs, making CCL21 a likely candidate to attract or retain CCR7-expressing tumor cells to or within LNs [18].

In a murine model of melanoma, CCR7-overexpressing B16 melanoma cells (CCR7-B16) metastasized with much higher frequency to tumor-draining LN compared to control B16 cells that did not express CCR7 [20]. Moreover, inhibition of CCL21 with neutralizing antibodies blocked LN metastasis following inoculation of CCR7-B16 cells in peripheral tissues [20]. These results suggested the expression of CCR7 was sufficient to augment nodal metastasis by melanoma cells.

The association of CCR7 expression with LN metastasis was demonstrated in a variety of other solid tumors as well as in hematopoietic malignancy as described below. In the majority of those studies, a large number of primary and metastatic tumors were retrospectively analyzed for CCR7 protein expression by immunohistochemistry and/or for CCR7 mRNA expression by quantitative real-time PCR. Following analysis, CCR7 expression was statistically evaluated for its association with other clinical features besides nodal metastasis, including lymphatic invasion, primary tumor size, relapse-free survival, and overall survival.

CCR7 expression was positively correlated with regional LN metastasis in T1 breast cancer [21], cervical cancer [22], melanoma [23], colorectal carcinoma [24], gastric carcinoma [25, 26], oral and oropharyngeal squamous cell carcinoma [27], squamous cell carcinoma of tonsil [28], esophageal squamous cell carcinoma [29], squamous cell carcinoma of the head and neck (SCCHN) [30], thyroid carcinoma [31], nonsmall cell lung cancer [32], hepatocellular cancer [33], prostate cancer [34], adult T-cell leukemia [35], and chronic lymphocytic leukemia [36, 37].

In addition to enhanced nodal metastasis, CCR7 expression was significantly higher in patients with cervical cancer showing larger tumor size, deeper stromal invasion and vaginal invasion, and lymph-vascular space involvement. Moreover, the disease-free survival and overall survival rates of patients that expressed both CXCR4 and CCR7 were significantly reduced [22]. Analysis of primary melanomas revealed a significant correlation of CCR7 expression with Breslow thickness, the depth of penetration of the tumor into the skin [23]. CCR7 expression was also significantly linked to decreased survival in patients with colon cancer [24]. CCR7 expression was significantly higher in patients with gastric carcinoma that exhibited larger tumor size, deeper invasion, higher rates of lymphatic invasion, more venous invasion, advanced disease stage, and worse surgical outcomes [25, 26].

CCR7 expression was also highly correlated with reduced disease-free and overall survival, more progressive stages, higher rates of local recurrence, and cancer death in patients with oral and oropharyngeal squamous cell carcinoma [27]. Analysis of patients with tonsillar squamous cell carcinoma revealed a significant correlation between high levels of CCR7 expression and decreased relapse-free, disease-specific, and overall survival [28]. High levels of CCR7 expression were significantly correlated with lymphatic invasion, tumor depth, disease stage, and poor survival in patients with esophageal squamous cell carcinoma [29]. CCR7 expression was also significantly linked with disease stage and lymphatic invasion in patients with nonsmall cell lung cancer [32]. In addition, CCR7, together with STX1A and HIF1A, have been classified as prognostic markers to predict overall survival rate in nonsmall cell lung cancer patients in a stage-independent manner [38]. A strong correlation of CCR7 expression with progressed local tumors was also found in patients with hepatocellular carcinoma [33]. In patients with axillary node-positive primary breast cancer, the expression of CCR7 was associated with increased risk of relapse of skin metastasis [39].

Overall, CCR7 upregulation in many human cancers not only enhances LN metastasis, but also correlates with larger primary tumors, deeper lymphatic invasion, more progressed cancer stage, and poor survival.

Mechanisms that Promote CCR7 Upregulation in Human Cancers

Even though abundant evidence convincingly shows the correlation of high levels of CCR7 expression by many human cancers with nodal metastasis and poor prognosis, there have been only a few reports that have elucidated the underlying mechanisms that lead to the upregulation of CCR7 by primary tumor cells.

In human breast tumor cell lines, endothelins have been reported to induce CCR7 expression at both mRNA level and protein level through activation of endothelin receptor A (ET-RA) in a hypoxia-inducible factor-1α (HIF-1α)-dependent manner [40]. The endothelin system includes three small 21-amino acid peptides ligands (ET-1, ET-2, and ET-3), two G-protein-coupled receptors (ET-RA and ET-RB), and two activating peptidases [41]. Increased expression of endothelins and their receptors was found in invasive breast cancer compared to normal breast tissues or benign fibroadenomas [42, 43]. In human primary breast cancer, endothelin expression was correlated with CCR7 expression, both of which were associated with LN metastasis [40].

Endothelins and their receptors may be induced within the tumor microenvironment by hypoxia via stabilization of HIF-1α as well as by inflammatory cytokines and chemokines [44]. These studies imply that multiple factors within the tumor microenvironment upregulate endothelin expression in local tumor regions, which in turn induces CCR7 expression by tumor cells. Interestingly, another chemokine receptor (i.e., CXCR4) associated with cancer cells is also induced by hypoxia via HIF-1-dependent mechanisms [19], suggesting that hypoxia may be an inducer of a variety of chemokine receptors. (See Chapter 3.)

In human melanoma cell lines, epigenetic changes may be involved in the upregulation of functional CCR7 expression [45]. Histone and chromatin modifications including acetylation, phosphorylation, methylation, and/or ubiquitylation are correlated with gene silencing or gene activation. Among those modifications, histone deacetylation and DNA methylation often repress gene transcription. Treating human melanoma cell lines with a histone deacetylation inhibitor, trichostatin A (TSA), significantly increased CCR7 expression, which was further enhanced by a demethylating reagent, 5-Aza-2-deoxycytidine (5-Aza) [45]. Histone deacetylation inhibitors and DNA methylation inhibitors alone or in combination have been tested in several clinical trials to treat different malignant tumors [46, 47]. However, these reagents may paradoxically enhance the expression of chemokine receptors, leading to enhanced cancer metastases. Therefore, using these reagents in anticancer therapy should be carefully evaluated.

Effects of CCR7 Expression on Cancer Cell Chemotaxis, Invasion, and Tumor Formation

In general, chemokines activate several signaling pathways after engagement with their cognate G-protein-coupled receptors, including phosphatidylinositol 3-kinase (PI3K), phospholipase C (PLC), RAS and RHO (RAS homolog) family small GTPase, and mitogen-activated protein kinase (MAPK) signaling cascades [48, 49] (Fig. 1). CCL21 (at high concentrations) has also been reported to inhibit T-cell proliferation by delaying degradation of the cyclin-dependent kinase inhibitor, p27(Kip1), and downmodulating CDK1 [17].

Reorganization of the actin cytoskeleton is an early downstream event in the migratory response to chemokines, followed by the formation of pseudopodia, which is required for the invasion of malignant cells into the tissues and eventual metastasis formation [50]. Not surprisingly, signaling through CCR7 by treatment with CCL19 or CCL21 triggered rapid intracellular actin polymerization, pseudopodia formation, and enhanced migration and invasion in vitro in human breast cancer cells, metastatic SCCHN cells, a thyroid tumor cell line (TPC-1), and esophageal carcinoma cell lines [18, 29, 31, 51].

Stimulation of leukocytes with chemokines has long been known to activate $\beta1$ and $\beta2$ integrins, which mediate firm adhesion of leukocytes onto endothelial cells of the vessel wall before they migrate into the tissues [52]. Evidence of chemokine-mediated activation of integrins has also been observed in B16 melanoma cells that overexpressed the CXCR4 receptor [53]. Ligation of the CXCR4 receptor in B16 melanoma cells also increased expression of matrix metalloproteinases (MMPs), a group of enzymes that degrade the major structural protein components of the extracellular matrix and basement membrane. Such activation of MMPs within the tumor microenvironment has been linked with tumor progression and metastasis [54]. In addition, stimulating TPC-1 cells with

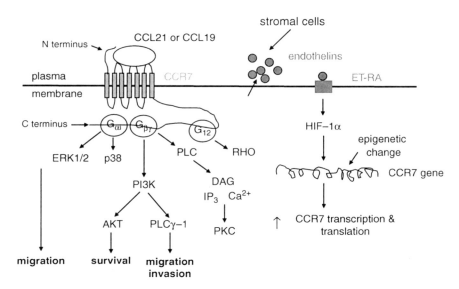

Fig. 1 CCR7 signaling pathways and CCR7 upregulation in tumor cells. Upon stimulation by CCL19 or CCL21, $\beta\gamma$ subunits of G protein are dissociated from $G\alpha_i$ subunit. $\beta\gamma$ subunits activate phospholipase C (PLC) and phosphatidylinositol 3 kinase (PI3K) pathways, whereas $G\alpha_i$ subunit directly activates mitogen-activated protein kinase (MAPK) signaling cascades. Distinct signaling pathways downstream of CCR7 are responsible for migration, invasion, and survival of tumor cells as indicated in the figure. Both tumor cells and stromal cells within tumor microenvironment can secrete endothelins, which induce CCR7 expression by tumor cells at both mRNA and protein levels through activation of endothelin receptor A (ET-RA) and stabilization of hypoxia-inducible factor-1α (HIF-1α). Epigenetic changes have also been implied in inducing CCR7 expression by tumor cells

CCL21 promoted β1-integrin expression and MMP-2/MMP-9 secretion as well as TPC-1 cell proliferation [31]. CCL21 also induced $\alpha4\beta1$ integrin-dependent adhesion of human nonsmall cell lung cancer cell line to VCAM-1 [55].

There have been very few studies focused on CCR7 signaling pathways that mediate migration and invasion of tumor cells in vitro. Activation of CCR7 by CCL19 stimulated chemotaxis and invasion of SCCHN cells, which was dependent on activation of PI3K and its downstream substrate PLCγ-1, but not the Akt (protein kinase B) pathway [51]. CCL21/CCR7 interaction also induced MMP-9 secretion and migration through Matrigel by B cell chronic lymphocytic leukemia cells in an ERK1/2/c-Fos pathway-dependent manner [56].

Chemokine receptors also activate key prosurvival pathways, including PI3K and its downstream effector, Akt. Murakami et al. have shown that CCR10-overexpressing B16 melanoma cells that were treated with CCL27 acquire rapid resistance to killing by tumor antigen-specific CD8 T cells in vitro. They subsequently showed that the PI3K pathway was critical for the acquisition of resistance to killing by demonstrating that wortmannin-treated CCR10-B16 cells were sensitive to killing by tumor-specific T cells [57]. In vivo, they showed that CCR10-expressing B16 cells could form tumors in mouse ear skin whereas control B16 cells could not. In this system, host immunity clearly played a role in preventing tumor formation in the control cells since tumors formed equally well in immunodeficient mice. Lastly, functional inhibition of skin-derived CCL27 with neutralizing antibodies prevented CCR10-B16 melanoma tumor formation.

Recently, we have demonstrated that, in addition to stimulating LN metastasis, CCR7 overexpression by B16 cells also facilitates tumorigenesis following cutaneous implantation (Fig. 2) [58]. Interestingly, serial measurements of nodal metastasis indicated that large numbers of metastatic B16 cells did not accumulate in the LN until CCR7-B16 skin tumors were grossly visible. Messenger RNA signal for CCL21 was easily detectable in the skin, perhaps originating from lymphatic endothelial cells that are known to constitutively synthesize this chemokine [59]. Thus, CCR7 apparently enhances nodal metastasis at a relatively late stage in tumor development in this model [58].

These data suggest that a number of chemokine receptors, including CCR7, activate prosurvival signals and facilitate tumor formation by cancer cells. Signaling through PI3K and its downstream mediator, Akt, is likely to be important since one outcome is protection of cancer cells from killing by host immune cells. Inhibition of chemokine receptor-mediated signaling may not be sufficient to kill cancer cells as a single therapy, but recent evidence suggests that combining chemokine receptor antagonists with specific antitumor therapy may be synergistic in efficacy [60].

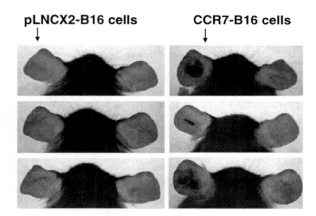

Fig. 2 Overexpression of CCR7 in B16 permits tumor formation following cutaneous implantation. 1×10^5 B16 murine melanoma cells that had been retrovirally transduced with either CCR7 cDNA or with vector (pLNCX2) only were injected (as indicated with *arrow*) into the left ear skin of mice just above the plane of the ear cartilage. Mice were photographed 20 days following inoculation with all ($n=20$) CCR10-B16-injected mice forming tumors whereas only 2 of 20 vector-B16 cell-injected mice formed tumors (3 of 20 mice from each group are shown). In these and subsequent similar experiments, nearly all mice injected with CCR7-B16 cells developed gross LN metastases whereas mice injected with control cells did not form nodal metastases

Mechanisms of Tumor Cell Homing to Lymphatics

Clinical as well as experimental data have strongly suggested that expression of CCR7 facilitates tumor cell metastasis to LN, particularly those draining the primary tumor site. Since CCR7 ligands are constitutively expressed by lymphatic, as opposed to vascular, endothelial cells [59, 61], it is reasonable to speculate that tumor-derived factors that increase the formation of lymphatic vessels will result in an increased probability of migration and/or invasion of tumor cells into vessels that constitutively produce CCL21 or CCL19. Studies have shown that tumor cells secrete lymphatic endothelial growth factors such as vascular endothelial growth factor C (VEGF-C) and VEGF-D to induce migration and growth of intratumoral lymphatic vessels (lymphangiogenesis). Expression (and overexpression) of VEGF-C and -D have been determined to enhance metastasis to regional LNs in experimental tumor models [62, 63, 64, 65]. Increased numbers of larger lymphatic vessels were detected in human metastatic melanoma samples compared to nonmetastatic samples [66, 67]. The presence of increased intratumoral lymphatic vessels and necessity of lymphangiogenesis, however, for lymphatic metastasis in human cancers remain controversial [68, 69, 70].

Autocrine expression of CCL19 or CCL21 by tumors may be a novel mechanism by which these chemokines contribute to lymphatic metastasis. Shields et al. have shown that several different CCR7-expressing tumor cell lines secrete high levels of CCL19 and CCL21, particularly in a 3D environment compared to 2D culture. These CCR7 ligands formed transcellular gradients that stimulated lymphatic-independent migration under the influence of slow interstitial flow [71]. These authors found that the combination of lymphatic-produced chemokine in addition to the transcellular gradient derived from autologous production of chemokines resulted in a synergistic increase in tumor cell migration toward lymphatic vessels.

Effects of CCR7 Expression by CD8 T Cells and Mature DCs in Cancer Immunotherapy

Tumor-reactive CD8$^+$ T cells are critical cancer-fighting components of the immune system. Upon encounter with antigens, naïve CD8 T cells proliferate and differentiate through early, intermediate, and late effector stages depending on the strength of T-cell receptor and ancillary signaling [72]. Differentiation from an early stage to late stage of effector CD8 T cells is characterized by progressive downregulation of CD62L, CCR7, β7 integrin, and CD27 and the concurrent upregulation of CD44, CD69, CD25, granzyme B, and perforin [73].

Circulating CD8$^+$CCR7$^+$ T cells (early effectors) isolated from patients with SCCHN as well as healthy donors were protected from spontaneous and induced apoptosis upon stimulation by CCL19 or CCL21, when compared to circulating $CD8^+CCR7^-$ T cells (late effectors). This was achieved through activation of PI3K/AKT pathway and subsequent upregulation of Bcl-2 expression. CCR7 expression by CD8 T cells was also correlated with low levels of pro-apoptotic Bax and Fas expression. However, the percentage of circulating $CD8^+CCR7^+$ T cells was significantly reduced in cancer patients and was replaced by apoptosis-sensitive $CD8^+CCR7^-$ T cells compared to healthy donors [74], suggesting a dysregulated lymphocyte homeostasis in cancer patients that may have a diminished antitumor immune response.

Preconditioning refractory metastatic melanoma patients with a lymphodepleting regimen followed by infusion of in vitro expanded autologous tumor infiltrating lymphocytes (TILs) has achieved objective clinical responses in ~50% of patients [75]. In a murine model of adoptive therapy that utilizes melanoma antigen-specific, transgenic T cells to treat established B16 melanoma tumors, activated pmel-1 $CD8^+$ T cells acquired terminally differentiated effector properties after multiple rounds of in vitro stimulation with antigen and IL-2. These T cells showed increased cytolytic activity and higher levels of IFN-γ production compared to T cells that had been exposed to fewer rounds of stimulation. However, when adoptively transferred into lymphodepleted B16 tumor-bearing WT mice, terminally differentiated pmel-1 CD8 T cells were at least 100-fold less effective than early effector CD8 cells in antitumor efficacy [73]. This finding poses new challenge for adoptive cell transfer (ACT)-based immunotherapy that expands TIL clones extensively in vitro, inevitably leading to the selection of $CD62L^-CCR7^-$ late-stage or terminally differentiated TIL clones for adoptive transfer [76]. Thus, balancing the quality and quantity of the transferred cells seems crucial in improving clinical outcome of ACT therapy for cancer. Development of TIL expansion protocols that selectively increase CCR7 expression may be useful in increasing the "quality" of the T cells prior to adoptive transfer in cancer patients.

DC-based immunotherapy that immunizes cancer patients with autologous DCs loaded ex vivo with tumor antigens has been vigorously pursued with the goal of stimulating endogenous host antitumor immune responses [77]. Autologous DCs are commonly generated from peripheral blood-derived monocytes and undergo a maturation process in vitro that upregulates CCR7 expression (and thus enhances LN migration capacity). Beyond simply increasing the ability of DC to chemotactically migrate to lymphatic vessels, CCR7 expression may protect mature DCs from apoptosis through activation of PI3K and AKT1 pathway [78]. The extended longevity of DCs within lymphoid tissues may increase their probability of eliciting an effective immune response against tumors.

Only a small percentage (<1%), however, of adoptively transferred DCs in patients reaches regional LNs [79]. Okada et al. have attempted to circumvent this problem by transducing tumor antigen-loaded DC with CCR7 (CCR7-DCs). When injected intradermally into mice, CCR7-DCs migrated into the draining LNs 5.5-fold more efficiently than control DCs. CCR7-DCs cotransduced with gp100, a melanoma-specific antigen, significantly delayed the growth of B16 melanoma in WT mice compared to DCs transduced with gp100 alone [80]. These results suggest that manipulating CCR7 expression by DCs may alter their trafficking and/or survival properties in order to increase their antitumor efficacy.

Summary

Since 2001, the association of CCR7 expression by tumor cells with LN metastasis (and associated poor clinical outcome) has been validated in a large number of solid tumors as well as in hematopoietic malignancies. Our recent data indicate that CCR7 may also be directly involved in tumor formation or in protecting tumors from killing by host immune cells. Local factors such as hypoxia, cytokines (endothelins), or epigenetic changes may be involved in the upregulation of CCR7 by tumor cells. Through distinct signaling pathways, activation of CCR7 by its cognate ligands, CCL21 or CCL19, promotes migration, invasion, and proliferation of tumor cells in vitro. In addition to responding to exogenous sources of CCR7 ligands, CCR7-expressing tumor cells facilitate their own migration toward CCL21-expressing lymphatics by generating transcellular gradients of CCL19/21. While CCR7 antagonists appear to block LN metastasis in short-term experimental models, the dual roles of CCR7 in protective immunity and tolerance suggest that these agents must be carefully evaluated. Meanwhile, increasing CCR7 expression in DCs may represent a potentially useful means of improving the efficacy of in vivo DC vaccination strategies.

References

1. Sanchez-Sanchez, N., L. Riol-Blanco, and J. L. Rodriguez-Fernandez. 2006. The multiple personalities of the chemokine receptor CCR7 in dendritic cells. *J Immunol* 176:5153–5159.
2. Saeki, H., A. M. Moore, M. J. Brown, and S. T. Hwang. 1999. Cutting edge: secondary lymphoid-tissue chemokine (SLC) and CC chemokine receptor 7 (CCR7) participate in the emigration pathway of mature dendritic cells from the skin to regional lymph nodes. *J Immunol* 162:2472–2475.
3. Forster, R., A. Schubel, D. Breitfeld, E. Kremmer, I. Renner-Muller, E. Wolf, and M. Lipp. 1999. CCR7 coordinates the primary immune response by establishing functional microenvironments in secondary lymphoid organs. *Cell* 99:23–33.
4. Schneider, M. A., J. G. Meingassner, M. Lipp, H. D. Moore, and A. Rot. 2007. CCR7 is required for the in vivo function of CD4+ CD25+ regulatory T cells. *The Journal of experimental medicine* 204:735–745.
5. Worbs, T., and R. Forster. 2007. A key role for CCR7 in establishing central and peripheral tolerance. *Trends Immunol* 28:274–280.
6. Yoshida, R., M. Nagira, M. Kitaura, N. Imagawa, T. Imai, and O. Yoshie. 1998. Secondary lymphoid-tissue chemokine is a functional ligand for the CC chemokine receptor CCR7. *J Biol Chem* 273:7118–7122.

7. Nagira, M., T. Imai, K. Hieshima, J. Kusuda, M. Ridanpaa, S. Takagi, M. Nishimura, M. Kakizaki, H. Nomiyama, and O. Yoshie. 1997. Molecular cloning of a novel human CC chemokine secondary lymphoid-tissue chemokine that is a potent chemoattractant for lymphocytes and mapped to chromosome 9p13. *J Biol Chem* 272:19518–19524.

8. Hedrick, J. A., and A. Zlotnik. 1997. Identification and characterization of a novel beta chemokine containing six conserved cysteines. *J Immunol* 159:1589–1593.

9. Gunn, M. D., K. Tangemann, C. Tam, J. G. Cyster, S. D. Rosen, and L. T. Williams. 1998. A chemokine expressed in lymphoid high endothelial venules promotes the adhesion and chemotaxis of naive T lymphocytes. *Proc Natl Acad Sci U S A* 95:258–263.

10. Yoshida, R., T. Imai, K. Hieshima, J. Kusuda, M. Baba, M. Kitaura, M. Nishimura, M. Kakizaki, H. Nomiyama, and O. Yoshie. 1997. Molecular cloning of a novel human CC chemokine EBI1-ligand chemokine that is a specific functional ligand for EBI1, CCR7. *J Biol Chem* 272:13803–13809.

11. Rossi, D. L., A. P. Vicari, K. Franz-Bacon, T. K. McClanahan, and A. Zlotnik. 1997. Identification through bioinformatics of two new macrophage proinflammatory human chemokines: MIP-3alpha and MIP-3beta. *J Immunol* 158:1033–1036.

12. Ngo, V. N., H. L. Tang, and J. G. Cyster. 1998. Epstein-Barr virus-induced molecule 1 ligand chemokine is expressed by dendritic cells in lymphoid tissues and strongly attracts naive T cells and activated B cells. *J Exp Med* 188:181–191.

13. Sallusto, F., D. Lenig, R. Forster, M. Lipp, A. Lanzavecchia. 1999. Two subsets of memory T lymphocytes with distinct homing potentials and effector functions. *Nature* 401:708–712.

14. Campbell, J. J., J. Hedrick, A. Zlotnik, M. A. Siani, D. A. Thompson, and E. C. Butcher. 1998. Chemokines and the arrest of lymphocytes rolling under flow conditions. *Science* 279:381–384.

15. Gunn, M. D., S. Kyuwa, C. Tam, T. Kakiuchi, A. Matsuzawa, L. T. Williams, and H. Nakano. 1999. Mice lacking expression of secondary lymphoid organ chemokine have defects in lymphocyte homing and dendritic cell localization. *J Exp Med* 189:451–460.

16. Ziegler, E., F. Gueler, S. Rong, M. Mengel, O. Witzke, A. Kribben, H. Haller, U. Kunzendorf, and S. Krautwald. 2006. CCL19-IgG prevents allograft rejection by impairment of immune cell trafficking. *J Am Soc Nephrol* 17:2521–2532.

17. Ziegler, E., M. Oberbarnscheidt, S. Bulfone-Paus, R. Forster, U. Kunzendorf, and S. Krautwald. 2007. CCR7 signaling inhibits T cell proliferation. *J Immunol* 179:6485–6493.

18. Muller, A., B. Homey, H. Soto, N. Ge, D. Catron, M. E. Buchanan, T. McClanahan, E. Murphy, W. Yuan, S. N. Wagner, J. L. Barrera, A. Mohar, E. Verastegui, and A. Zlotnik. 2001. Involvement of chemokine receptors in breast cancer metastasis. *Nature* 410:50–56.

19. Kakinuma, T., and S. T. Hwang. 2006. Chemokines, chemokine receptors, and cancer metastasis. *J Leukoc Biol* 79:639–651.

20. Wiley, H. E., E. B. Gonzalez, W. Maki, M. T. Wu, and S. T. Hwang. 2001. Expression of CC chemokine receptor-7 and regional lymph node metastasis of B16 murine melanoma. *J Natl Cancer Inst* 93:1638–1643.

21. Cabioglu, N., M. S. Yazici, B. Arun, K. R. Broglio, G. N. Hortobagyi, J. E. Price, and A. Sahin. 2005. CCR7 and CXCR4 as novel biomarkers predicting axillary lymph node metastasis in T1 breast cancer. *Clin Cancer Res* 11:5686–5693.

22. Kodama, J., Hasengaowa, T. Kusumoto, N. Seki, T. Matsuo, Y. Ojima, K. Nakamura, A. Hongo, and Y. Hiramatsu. 2007. Association of CXCR4 and CCR7 chemokine receptor expression and lymph node metastasis in human cervical cancer. *Ann Oncol* 18:70–76.

23. Takeuchi, H., A. Fujimoto, M. Tanaka, T. Yamano, E. Hsueh, and D. S. Hoon. 2004. CCL21 chemokine regulates chemokine receptor CCR7 bearing malignant melanoma cells. *Clin Cancer Res* 10:2351–2358.

24. Gunther, K., J. Leier, G. Henning, A. Dimmler, R. Weissbach, W. Hohenberger, and R. Forster. 2005. Prediction of lymph node metastasis in colorectal carcinoma by expression of chemokine receptor CCR7. *Int J Cancer* 116:726–733.

25. Ishigami, S., S. Natsugoe, A. Nakajo, K. Tokuda, Y. Uenosono, T. Arigami, M. Matsumoto, H. Okumura, S. Hokita, and T. Aikou. 2007. Prognostic value of CCR7 expression in gastric cancer. *Hepatogastroenterology* 54:1025–1028.

26. Yan, C., Z. G. Zhu, Y. Y. Yu, J. Ji, Y. Zhang, Y. B. Ji, M. Yan, J. Chen, B. Y. Liu, H. R. Yin, and Y. Z. Lin. 2004. Expression of vascular endothelial growth factor C and chemokine receptor CCR7 in gastric carcinoma and their values in predicting lymph node metastasis. *World J Gastroenterol* 10:783–790.

27. Tsuzuki, H., N. Takahashi, A. Kojima, N. Narita, H. Sunaga, T. Takabayashi, and S. Fujieda. 2006. Oral and oropharyngeal squamous cell carcinomas expressing CCR7 have poor prognoses. *Auris Nasus Larynx* 33:37–42.

28. Pitkin, L., S. Luangdilok, C. Corbishley, P. O. Wilson, P. Dalton, D. Bray, S. Mady, P. Williamson, T. Odutoye, P. Rhys Evans, K. N. Syrigos, C. M. Nutting, Y. Barbachano, S. Eccles, and K. J. Harrington. 2007. Expression of CC chemokine receptor 7 in tonsillar cancer predicts cervical nodal metastasis, systemic relapse and survival. *Br J Cancer* 97:670–677.

29. Ding, Y., Y. Shimada, M. Maeda, A. Kawabe, J. Kaganoi, I. Komoto, Y. Hashimoto, M. Miyake, H. Hashida, and M. Imamura. 2003. Association of CC chemokine receptor 7 with lymph node metastasis of esophageal squamous cell carcinoma. *Clin Cancer Res* 9:3406–3412.

30. Wang, J., L. Xi, J. L. Hunt, W. Gooding, T. L. Whiteside, Z. Chen, T. E. Godfrey, and R. L. Ferris. 2004. Expression pattern of chemokine receptor 6 (CCR6) and CCR7 in squamous cell carcinoma of the head and neck identifies a novel metastatic phenotype. *Cancer Res* 64:1861–1866.

31. Sancho, M., J. M. Vieira, C. Casalou, M. Mesquita, T. Pereira, B. M. Cavaco, S. Dias, and V. Leite. 2006. Expression and function of the chemokine receptor CCR7 in thyroid carcinomas. *J Endocrinol* 191:229–238.

32. Takanami, I. 2003. Overexpression of CCR7 mRNA in nonsmall cell lung cancer: correlation with lymph node metastasis. *Int J Cancer* 105:186–189.

33. Schimanski, C. C., R. Bahre, I. Gockel, T. Junginger, N. Simiantonaki, S. Biesterfeld, T. Achenbach, T. Wehler, P. R. Galle, and M. Moehler. 2006. Chemokine receptor CCR7 enhances intrahepatic and lymphatic dissemination of human hepatocellular cancer. *Oncol Rep* 16:109–113.

34. Heresi, G. A., J. Wang, R. Taichman, J. A. Chirinos, J. J. Regalado, D. M. Lichtstein, and J. D. Rosenblatt. 2005. Expression of the chemokine receptor CCR7 in prostate cancer presenting with generalized lymphadenopathy: report of a case, review of the literature, and analysis of chemokine receptor expression. *Urol Oncol* 23:261–267.

35. Hasegawa, H., T. Nomura, M. Kohno, N. Tateishi, Y. Suzuki, N. Maeda, R. Fujisawa, O. Yoshie, and S. Fujita. 2000. Increased chemokine receptor CCR7/EBI1 expression enhances the infiltration of lymphoid organs by adult T-cell leukemia cells. *Blood* 95:30–38.

36. Till, K. J., K. Lin, M. Zuzel, and J. C. Cawley. 2002. The chemokine receptor CCR7 and alpha4 integrin are important for migration of chronic lymphocytic leukemia cells into lymph nodes. *Blood* 99:2977–2984.

37. Lopez-Giral, S., N. E. Quintana, M. Cabrerizo, M. Alfonso-Perez, M. Sala-Valdes, V. G. De Soria, J. M. Fernandez-Ranada, E. Fernandez-Ruiz, and C. Munoz. 2004. Chemokine receptors that mediate B cell homing to secondary lymphoid tissues are highly expressed in B cell chronic lymphocytic leukemia and non-Hodgkin lymphomas with widespread nodular dissemination. *J Leukoc Biol* 76:462–471.

38. Lau, S. K., P. C. Boutros, M. Pintilie, F. H. Blackhall, C. Q. Zhu, D. Strumpf, M. R. Johnston, G. Darling, S. Keshavjee, T. K. Waddell, N. Liu, D. Lau, L. Z. Penn, F. A. Shepherd, I. Jurisica, S. D. Der, and M. S. Tsao. 2007. Three-gene prognostic classifier for early-stage non small-cell lung cancer. *J Clin Oncol* 25:5562–5569.

39. Andre, F., N. Cabioglu, H. Assi, J. C. Sabourin, S. Delaloge, A. Sahin, K. Broglio, J. P. Spano, C. Combadiere, C. Bucana, J. C. Soria, and M. Cristofanilli. 2006. Expression of chemokine receptors predicts the site of metastatic relapse in patients with axillary node positive primary breast cancer. *Ann Oncol* 17:945–951.
40. Wilson, J. L., J. Burchell, and M. J. Grimshaw. 2006. Endothelins induce CCR7 expression by breast tumor cells via endothelin receptor A and hypoxia-inducible factor-1. *Cancer Res* 66:11802–11807.
41. Kedzierski, R. M., and M. Yanagisawa. 2001. Endothelin system: the double-edged sword in health and disease. *Annu Rev Pharmacol Toxicol* 41:851–876.
42. Alanen, K., D. X. Deng, and S. Chakrabarti. 2000. Augmented expression of endothelin-1, endothelin-3 and the endothelin-B receptor in breast carcinoma. *Histopathology* 36:161–167.
43. Grimshaw, M. J., T. Hagemann, A. Ayhan, C. E. Gillett, C. Binder, and F. R. Balkwill. 2004. A role for endothelin-2 and its receptors in breast tumor cell invasion. *Cancer Res* 64:2461–2468.
44. Grimshaw, M. J. 2005. Endothelins in breast tumour cell invasion. *Cancer Lett* 222:129–138.
45. Mori, T., J. Kim, T. Yamano, H. Takeuchi, S. Huang, N. Umetani, K. Koyanagi, and D. S. Hoon. 2005. Epigenetic up-regulation of C-C chemokine receptor 7 and C-X-C chemokine receptor 4 expression in melanoma cells. *Cancer Res* 65:1800–1807.
46. Kelly, W. K., O. A. O'Connor, and P. A. Marks. 2002. Histone deacetylase inhibitors: from target to clinical trials. *Expert Opin Investig Drugs* 11:1695–1713.
47. Dowell, J. E., and J. D. Minna. 2004. Cancer chemotherapy targeted at reactivating the expression of epigenetically inactivated genes. *J Clin Oncol* 22:1353–1355.
48. Marinissen, M. J., and J. S. Gutkind. 2001. G-protein-coupled receptors and signaling networks: emerging paradigms. *Trends Pharmacol Sci* 22:368–376.
49. Kinashi, T. 2005. Intracellular signalling controlling integrin activation in lymphocytes. *Nat Rev Immunol* 5:546–559.
50. Verschueren, H., I. Van der Taelen, J. Dewit, J. De Braekeleer, and P. De Baetselier. 1994. Metastatic competence of BW5147 T-lymphoma cell lines is correlated with in vitro invasiveness, motility and F-actin content. *J Leukoc Biol* 55:552–556.
51. Wang, J., X. Zhang, S. M. Thomas, J. R. Grandis, A. Wells, Z. G. Chen, and R. L. Ferris. 2005. Chemokine receptor 7 activates phosphoinositide-3 kinase-mediated invasive and prosurvival pathways in head and neck cancer cells independent of EGFR. *Oncogene* 24:5897–5904.
52. Baggiolini, M. 1998. Chemokines and leukocyte traffic. *Nature* 392:565–568.
53. Cardones, A. R., T. Murakami, and S. T. Hwang. 2003. CXCR4 enhances adhesion of B16 tumor cells to endothelial cells in vitro and in vivo via beta (1) integrin. *Cancer Res* 63:6751–6757.
54. Overall, C. M., and C. Lopez-Otin. 2002. Strategies for MMP inhibition in cancer: innovations for the post-trial era. *Nat Rev Cancer* 2:657–672.
55. Koizumi, K., Y. Kozawa, Y. Ohashi, E. S. Nakamura, Y. Aozuka, H. Sakurai, K. Ichiki, Y. Doki, T. Misaki, and I. Saiki. 2007. CCL21 promotes the migration and adhesion of highly lymph node metastatic human non-small cell lung cancer Lu-99 in vitro. *Oncol Rep* 17:1511–1516.
56. Redondo-Munoz, J., M. Jose Terol, J. A. Garcia-Marco, and A. Garcia-Pardo. 2008. Matrix metalloproteinase-9 is up-regulated by CCL21/CCR7 interaction via extracellular signal-regulated kinase-1/2 signaling and is involved in CCL21-driven B-cell chronic lymphocytic leukemia cell invasion and migration. *Blood* 111:383–386.
57. Murakami, T., A. R. Cardones, S. E. Finkelstein, N. P. Restifo, B. A. Klaunberg, F. O. Nestle, S. S. Castillo, P. A. Dennis, and S. T. Hwang. 2003. Immune evasion by murine melanoma mediated through CC chemokine receptor-10. *J Exp Med* 198:1337–1347.

58. Fang, L., V. Lee, E.Cha, H. Zhang, and S. T. Hwang. 2008. CCR7 regulates B16 murine melanoma cell tumorigenesis in skin. *J. Leukou Biol* 84(4):965–72.
59. Kriehuber, E., S. Breiteneder-Geleff, M. Groeger, A. Soleiman, S. F. Schoppmann, G. Stingl, D. Kerjaschki, and D. Maurer. 2001. Isolation and characterization of dermal lymphatic and blood endothelial cells reveal stable and functionally specialized cell lineages. *J Exp Med* 194:797–808.
60. Lee, C. H., T. Kakinuma, J. Wang, H. Zhang, D. C. Palmer, N. P. Restifo, and S. T. Hwang. 2006. Sensitization of B16 tumor cells with a CXCR4 antagonist increases the efficacy of immunotherapy for established lung metastases. *Mol Cancer Ther* 5:2592–2599.
61. Shields, J. D., M. S. Emmett, D. B. Dunn, K. D. Joory, L. M. Sage, H. Rigby, P. S. Mortimer, A. Orlando, J. R. Levick, and D. O. Bates. 2007. Chemokine-mediated migration of melanoma cells towards lymphatics–a mechanism contributing to metastasis. *Oncogene* 26:2997–3005.
62. Skobe, M., T. Hawighorst, D. G. Jackson, R. Prevo, L. Janes, P. Velasco, L. Riccardi, K. Alitalo, K. Claffey, and M. Detmar. 2001. Induction of tumor lymphangiogenesis by VEGF-C promotes breast cancer metastasis. *Nat Med* 7:192–198.
63. Stacker, S. A., C. Caesar, M. E. Baldwin, G. E. Thornton, R. A. Williams, R. Prevo, D. G. Jackson, S. Nishikawa, H. Kubo, and M. G. Achen. 2001. VEGF-D promotes the metastatic spread of tumor cells via the lymphatics. *Nat Med* 7:186–191.
64. Mandriota, S. J., L. Jussila, M. Jeltsch, A. Compagni, D. Baetens, R. Prevo, S. Banerji, J. Huarte, R. Montesano, D. G. Jackson, L. Orci, K. Alitalo, G. Christofori, and M. S. Pepper. 2001. Vascular endothelial growth factor-C-mediated lymphangiogenesis promotes tumour metastasis. *EMBO J* 20:672–682.
65. He, Y., I. Rajantie, K. Pajusola, M. Jeltsch, T. Holopainen, S. Yla-Herttuala, T. Harding, K. Jooss, T. Takahashi, and K. Alitalo. 2005. Vascular endothelial cell growth factor receptor 3-mediated activation of lymphatic endothelium is crucial for tumor cell entry and spread via lymphatic vessels. *Cancer Res* 65:4739–4746.
66. Dadras, S. S., T. Paul, J. Bertoncini, L. F. Brown, A. Muzikansky, D. G. Jackson, U. Ellwanger, C. Garbe, M. C. Mihm, and M. Detmar. 2003. Tumor lymphangiogenesis: a novel prognostic indicator for cutaneous melanoma metastasis and survival. *Am J Pathol* 162:1951–1960.
67. Shields, J. D., M. Borsetti, H. Rigby, S. J. Harper, P. S. Mortimer, J. R. Levick, A. Orlando, and D. O. Bates. 2004. Lymphatic density and metastatic spread in human malignant melanoma. *Br J Cancer* 90:693–700.
68. Williams, C. S., R. D. Leek, A. M. Robson, S. Banerji, R. Prevo, A. L. Harris, and D. G. Jackson. 2003. Absence of lymphangiogenesis and intratumoural lymph vessels in human metastatic breast cancer. *J Pathol* 200:195–206.
69. Sipos, B., M. Kojima, K. Tiemann, W. Klapper, M. L. Kruse, H. Kalthoff, B. Schniewind, J. Tepel, H. Weich, D. Kerjaschki, and G. Kloppel. 2005. Lymphatic spread of ductal pancreatic adenocarcinoma is independent of lymphangiogenesis. *J Pathol* 207:301–312.
70. Wong, S. Y., H. Haack, D. Crowley, M. Barry, R. T. Bronson, and R. O. Hynes. 2005. Tumor-secreted vascular endothelial growth factor-C is necessary for prostate cancer lymphangiogenesis, but lymphangiogenesis is unnecessary for lymph node metastasis. *Cancer Res* 65:9789–9798.
71. Shields, J. D., M. E. Fleury, C. Yong, A. A. Tomei, G. J. Randolph, and M. A. Swartz. 2007. Autologous chemotaxis as a mechanism of tumor cell homing to lymphatics via interstitial flow and autocrine CCR7 signaling. *Cancer Cell* 11:526–538.
72. Lanzavecchia, A., and F. Sallusto. 2002. Progressive differentiation and selection of the fittest in the immune response. *Nat Rev Immunol* 2:982–987.
73. Gattinoni, L., C. A. Klebanoff, D. C. Palmer, C. Wrzesinski, K. Kerstann, Z. Yu, S. E. Finkelstein, M. R. Theoret, S. A. Rosenberg, and N. P. Restifo. 2005. Acquisition of full effector function in vitro paradoxically impairs the in vivo antitumor efficacy of adoptively transferred CD8+ T cells. *J Clin Invest* 115:1616–1626.

74. Kim, J. W., R. L. Ferris, and T. L. Whiteside. 2005. Chemokine C receptor 7 expression and protection of circulating CD8+ T lymphocytes from apoptosis. *Clin Cancer Res* 11:7901–7910.
75. Dudley, M. E., J. R. Wunderlich, J. C. Yang, R. M. Sherry, S. L. Topalian, N. P. Restifo, R. E. Royal, U. Kammula, D. E. White, S. A. Mavroukakis, L. J. Rogers, G. J. Gracia, S. A. Jones, D. P. Mangiameli, M. M. Pelletier, J. Gea-Banacloche, M. R. Robinson, D. M. Berman, A. C. Filie, A. Abati, and S. A. Rosenberg. 2005. Adoptive cell transfer therapy following non-myeloablative but lymphodepleting chemotherapy for the treatment of patients with refractory metastatic melanoma. *J Clin Oncol* 23:2346–2357.
76. Powell, D. J., Jr., M. E. Dudley, P. F. Robbins, and S. A. Rosenberg. 2005. Transition of late-stage effector T cells to CD27+ CD28+ tumor-reactive effector memory T cells in humans after adoptive cell transfer therapy. *Blood* 105:241–250.
77. Gilboa, E. 2007. DC-based cancer vaccines. *J Clin Invest* 117:1195–1203.
78. Sanchez-Sanchez, N., L. Riol-Blanco, G. de la Rosa, A. Puig-Kroger, J. Garcia-Bordas, D. Martin, N. Longo, A. Cuadrado, C. Cabanas, A. L. Corbi, P. Sanchez-Mateos, and J. L. Rodriguez-Fernandez. 2004. Chemokine receptor CCR7 induces intracellular signaling that inhibits apoptosis of mature dendritic cells. *Blood* 104:619–625.
79. Morse, M. A., R. E. Coleman, G. Akabani, N. Niehaus, D. Coleman, and H. K. Lyerly. 1999. Migration of human dendritic cells after injection in patients with metastatic malignancies. *Cancer Res* 59:56–58.
80. Okada, N., N. Mori, R. Koretomo, Y. Okada, T. Nakayama, O. Yoshie, H. Mizuguchi, T. Hayakawa, S. Nakagawa, T. Mayumi, T. Fujita, and A. Yamamoto. 2005. Augmentation of the migratory ability of DC-based vaccine into regional lymph nodes by efficient CCR7 gene transduction. *Gene Ther* 12:129–139.

The CCL5/CCR5 Axis in Cancer

Gali Soria and Adit Ben-Baruch

Abstract The multifaceted roles of chemokines and of their receptors in physiological and pathological conditions have motivated researchers to analyze their involvement also in malignant diseases. This chapter focuses on CCL5 (RANTES) and its CCR5 receptor in cancer, describing their expression patterns, activities, and roles in several malignancies. Thus far, CCL5 and/or CCR5 have been detected in many hematological malignancies and in a large number of solid tumors; however, extensive studies on CCL5 and CCR5 were performed only in a limited number of cancers, including primarily multiple myeloma, breast cancer, and melanoma. This chapter discusses the major findings in these three specific malignancies, and addresses other cancers in which preliminary evidence was provided, including gastric cancer and ovarian cancer. In the framework of this chapter, we discuss the expression patterns of CCL5 and CCR5 in patients, their associations with disease course and experiments that were performed in animal model systems in order to decipher the roles of the CCL5/CCR5 axis in tumor growth and metastasis. In addition, we describe possible mechanisms mediating the activity of this pair in specific malignancies, and their effects on the tumor cells and on cells of the tumor microenvironment. Also, when it is of relevance, we consider the roles of other receptors for CCL5 (CCR1, CCR3) and of additional high-affinity chemotactic ligands for CCR5 (MIP-1α, CCL3; MIP-1β, CCL4). Taken together, the different studies suggest that even if the CCL5/CCR5 axis may have an anti-tumor potential under specific conditions, it turns into a detrimental entity in defined cancer diseases, such as multiple myeloma and breast cancer. Overall, CCL5/CCR5 may have major implications in cancer, and they should be considered as potential therapeutic targets for the limitation of specific malignant diseases.

A. Ben-Baruch (✉)
Department of Cell Research and Immunology, George S. Wise Faculty of Life Sciences, Tel Aviv University, Tel Aviv 69978, Israel
e-mail: aditbb@tauex.tau.ac.il

A.M. Fulton (ed.), *Chemokine Receptors in Cancer*, Cancer Drug Discovery and Development, DOI 10.1007/978-1-60327-267-4_7,
© Humana Press, a part of Springer Science+Business Media, LLC 2009

Introduction

Cancer development and progression are multifactorial processes, in which intrinsic properties of the tumor cells are joined by microenvironmental factors, together giving rise to a detrimental cascade of events that leads to malignancy. Of the different factors that regulate tumorigenesis and metastasis, major emphasis was put recently on chemokines and their receptors. Chemokines were found to play diverse roles in cancer: promalignancy potential was attributed to some, others were identified as factors with antitumorigenic properties, and specific chemokines were found to have divergent roles under different conditions [1–7]. Moreover, the involvement of each specific chemokine in tumor development and metastasis depends to a large extent on the tumor type and on the model systems, and reflects the equilibrium between the effects of the chemokine on the tumor cells and on cells of the tumor microenvironment.

Of the different members of the chemokine family and their receptors, the present chapter focuses on CCL5 (RANTES) and its CCR5 receptor, and on their roles in malignancy. CCL5, as a key regulator of T-cell migration to inflammatory sites, was thoroughly studied for its activities in the immunological context. The chemokine is considered mainly as an inflammatory mediator, directing the migration of T cells to damaged/infected sites, inducing T-cell costimulation, and possibly also T-cell proliferation. In addition, it was suggested that CCL5 regulates T-cell differentiation, a notion supported by findings showing that Th1 cells express CCR5 [8–10]. In addition to its prominent roles in T-cell regulation, CCR5 mediates cellular responses to CCL5 in other cell types that express the receptor, including monocytes and macrophages [9–12].

CCR5 is one of the three high-affinity receptors for CCL5, acting side by side with CCR1 and CCR3 [13, 14]. Of these three receptors, CCR5 is the best studied due to its involvement in HIV pathogenesis. In similarity to all other chemokine receptors, CCR5 is a seven-transmembrane G-protein-coupled receptor, mediating diverse signaling cascades in response to its ligands. CCR5 is a promiscuous receptor, binding with high-affinity CCL5, CCL3 (MIP-1α), and CCL4 (MIP-1β), all being associated with Th1 responses [8, 9]. In similarity to other chemokines and their receptors, it is believed that the ability of CCL5 to bind several receptors and the promiscuity of CCR5 for several chemotactic ligands allow fine tuning of chemokine responses, and guarantees the existence of backup mechanisms that come into effect when one of the constituents is not fully active [15, 16].

During the last decade, the study of CCL5 has expanded far beyond its functions in inflammation and regulation of T-cell activities. Primarily, the identification of CCR5 as a major co-receptor for HIV has led to extensive research in this direction. In addition, the prominent role of CCL5 in leukocyte chemoattraction has raised the possibility that CCL5 determines the type and levels of leukocyte infiltrates in tumors, and that it affects antitumor immunity.

These hypotheses have motivated investigators to characterize the involvement of CCL5 in malignant diseases, and further emphasis was put on CCR5 due to its major involvement in a large number of physiological and pathological conditions.

Examination of the studies that were performed on the CCL5/CCR5 axis in malignancy indicates that the two members of this pair are expressed in hematological malignancies and in a large number of solid tumors. Having the aim of providing insights into the roles of these two components in cancer, we herein describe their expression patterns and roles in specific malignancies. In addition, when appropriate, the chapter was extended beyond the CCL5/CCR5 limits, and includes information on CCR1 and CCR3 as additional high-affinity receptors for CCL5, and on CCL3 and CCL4 as other high-affinity ligands of CCR5.

Thus far, the findings in the literature indicate that the CCL5/CCR5 pair, and in specific cases other associated members of the family, affect malignancy in divergent manners. At times they are associated with inhibition of tumor growth but in most cases they promote tumorigenicity and metastasis. Of note, only in relatively rare occasions a definite connection was established between the CCL5/CCR5 axis and the course of the malignant disease. Accordingly, this chapter focuses on specific malignancies in which more concrete evidence was provided for the roles of CCL5/CCR5 in tumor development and/or progression, focusing primarily on MM and breast cancer. Findings in melanoma, gastric cancer and ovarian cancer are also discussed, as they provide preliminary description of the expression patterns and possible involvement of the CCL5/CCR5 axis in these diseases.

Obviously, there is a need to expand our understanding of the involvement of the CCL5/CCR5 pair in malignancy. Extensive research on specific cancer types is required in order to provide conclusive evidence regarding the role of this axis in each disease, and on its consideration as a potential target for therapeutical modalities aimed at limitation of specific malignancies.

The CCL5/CCR5 Axis in Hematological Malignancies: Multiple Myeloma

Many studies were published during the last several years on the expression of CCL5 and of CCR5 in hematological malignancies. The large variety of investigations addressed different types of leukemia and lymphoma and have primarily analyzed the expression of these two components by the tumor cells. Of the different hematological cancers, MM was the tumor type providing the most comprehensive view on the roles played by CCR5 and CCR1 in disease course, with major emphasis on their CCL3 ligand.

MM is a plasma cell malignancy, characterized by accumulation of plasmablast/plasma cells in the bone marrow. Being of a post germinal origin, MM cells have to re-enter the bone marrow, where interactions with the bone marrow microenvironment take place, leading to osteolysis and angiogenesis. Obviously, the processes involved in MM are complex and depend on many different factors. Of these, recent studies have illuminated the potential involvement of the chemokine CCL3 (and also of CCL4) and of its CCR5 and CCR1 receptors in MM.

The major source for CCL3 in MM is the tumor cells, and production of the chemokine was detected in MM cell lines and in freshly isolated MM cells [17–22]. CCL3 is overexpressed in MM patients, and MM cells from patients with multiple bone lesions secreted higher amounts of CCL3 (and CCL4) than those from patients with less-advanced bone involvement [17, 20, 22]. Moreover, elevated CCL3 serum levels correlated with bone resorption, with the extent of bone disease and with lower probability of 3-year survival in MM patients [23, 24].

Further indication of the promalignancy role of CCL3 in MM was provided by the finding that increased CCL3 levels were found in diseased mice, and that antisense inhibition of the chemokine led to reduced tumor burden and longer survival of mice [25]. CCL3 also promoted the metastatic spread of MM by inducing signaling pathways leading to increased survival and proliferation of MM cells [21, 26].

Looking more carefully at the roles of CCL3 in MM, it was shown that the chemokine supports osteolysis. In line with this possibility, CCL3 enhanced osteoclast formation and CCL3 inhibition blocked this process [17, 18, 20, 22–25, 27]. Moreover, mice engrafted with MM cells expressing lower CCL3 levels did not show lytic lesions, and these cells demonstrated reduced adherence to stroma marrow cells [25].

The observed CCL3-mediated effect requires the expression of its corresponding receptors by appropriate target cells. Indeed, the expression of CCR5 and CCR1 was detected in bone marrow stroma cells and in osteoclast precursors [17–19, 27]. The two receptors were found to mediate osteoclastogenesis and osteoclastic resorption; their inhibition by antagonists gave rise to partial blocking of these processes; and neutralizing antibodies to the receptors inhibited CCL3-induced formation of osteoclasts [17–19]. Furthermore, inhibition of CCR5 and primarily of CCR1, has led in vivo to reduction in osteolytic lesions, and to reduced MM-induced angiogenesis [19].

In addition to the expression of CCL3 receptors by osteoclast precursors and bone marrow stroma cells, several studies have shown the expression of CCR5 and CCR1 by MM cell lines and by cells derived from patients [17–19, 21, 28, 29]. Although the extent of receptor expression varied in the different investigations, substantial evidence supported the ability of these receptors to mediate processes that play important roles in MM. Specifically, different studies have analyzed the contribution of CCR1 and CCR5 to tumor cell migration in response to CCL3, and to homing of MM cells to the bone marrow. In vitro migration of MM cells to CCL3 and also to CCL5 was identified, and in the case of CCL3 it was found to depend on CCR5 [19, 21, 29]. Additional studies substantiated the roles of the two receptors in homing and invasion: antibodies to CCR1 and CCR5 inhibited the ability of CCL3 to induce β_1 integrin upre-gulation, as well as the adherence of MM cells to stroma cells [18], and the use of CCR5 and CCR1 antagonists indicated that it was primarily CCR5 that was responsible for the in vivo homing of MM cells to the bone marrow [19].

Overall, the current observations propose two major mechanisms by which CCL3, CCL5 and their receptors support MM progression: the first is the ability of MM-derived CCL3 to act on osteoclasts and promote osteoclastogen-esis, and the second is migration of MM cells to the bone marrow in a CCL3/CCL5–CCR5/CCR1-dependent manner. Therefore, it is becoming evident that in MM the CCL5/CCR5 pair, and its associated members, need to be seriously considered as potential therapeutic targets.

The CCL5/CCR5 Axis in Solid Tumors

The study of the CCL5/CCR5 pair in solid tumors has encompassed many different tumor types, including breast cancer, melanoma, gastric cancer, ovarian cancer, cervical cancer, colorectal cancer, pancreatic cancer, renal carcinoma, sarcomas, neuroblastoma, glioblastoma, and others. In some of these malignan-cies, the findings on the CCL5/CCR5 axis were sporadic or descriptive, with no overall conclusion on the roles played by the chemokine and its receptor in disease course. However, some of the malignancies were more thoroughly researched, with studies providing evidence mainly of promalignancy activities for this pair. Of these, the most comprehensive findings were obtained in breast cancer, and accordingly, major emphasis is given in this chapter to this malig-nancy. In addition, initial indications on the roles of the CCL5/CCR5 axis were provided in melanoma, gastric cancer, and ovarian cancer, to be discussed herein.

Breast Cancer

During the last several years, the expression of CCL5 was extensively analyzed in breast cancer patients. It was found that the chemokine is expressed by breast tumor cells residing in primary tumors, in regional lymph nodes and in meta-static sites, and in addition the chemokine was detected in interstitial fluids perfusing the tumor, in pleural effusions and in serum ([30–38] and A. Ben-Baruch et al., unpublished results). Although in breast tumors the major source for CCL5 is the tumor cells, the expression of the chemokine was also noted in infiltrating leukocytes that reside at the tumor site, and in mesenchymal stem cells that play a role in breast cancer metastasis [30, 39].

Further analysis indicated that the chemokine was expressed by unstimu-lated human and murine breast cancer cell lines [30, 40–48]. In line with the inflammatory nature of the chemokine, its release by the tumor cells was shown to be potently induced by pro-inflammatory cytokines that are highly expressed at breast tumor sites, such as tumor necrosis factor α (TNFα) and interferon γ (IFNγ) [40, 49].

In parallel to findings describing the expression patterns of CCL5 in breast cancer, different studies have analyzed its association with disease development and progression. The first evidence of a direct correlation between CCL5 expression and breast malignancy was provided by the study of Luboshits et al. [30]. This investigation found that CCL5 was highly expressed by breast cancer cells in primary tumors however, no expression, or minimal presence of the chemokine, was noted in normal breast epithelium in proximity to tumor cells or in healthy individuals ([30] and A. Ben-Baruch et al., unpublished results). These results indicated that the expression of CCL5 was acquired in the course of malignant transformation, suggesting that it is involved in breast cancer development.

Moreover, a role for CCL5 in breast cancer progression was also proposed, since increased incidence and expression levels of the chemokine by breast tumor cells were significantly associated with more advanced disease stage [30]. Also, increased levels of CCL5 were found in patients with disease progression, relapse, and/or metastasis, compared to patients in remission [31]. Additional analyses that were done by molecular profiling supported the association between CCL5 expression in breast tumors and aggressive disease, since CCL5 expression was upregulated in inflammatory breast cancer (IBC), a highly aggressive form of disease, as compared to non-IBC patients [33].

Taken together, these findings suggested that CCL5 promotes processes of breast cancer aggressiveness and progression. Accordingly, a recent study has indicated that CCL5 expression by breast tumor cells could be a valuable prognostic factor for detection of stage II breast cancer patients who are at risk for disease progression [32]. Importantly, combined analysis of CCL5 expression with the lack of estrogen receptor α improved the prognostic value of each of these two markers, suggesting that they could be used in conjunction for detection of patients at risk for breast cancer progression [32].

Overall, the above studies found a significant association between increased expression of CCL5 by breast tumor cells and advanced breast cancer, as well as with risk to progression. This has raised the possibility that CCL5 serum levels, if elevated in breast cancer patients, could have diagnostic and/or prognostic value. Three of the studies that addressed this issue indicated that CCL5 serum levels were elevated in breast cancer patients compared to healthy individuals [31, 36, 37]. Therefore, it is possible that CCL5 plasma levels could serve as a marker for active disease, and further research on the diagnostic value of CCL5 should be considered.

In parallel, some investigators have defined CCL5 serum levels in patients undergoing unique therapeutic regimens, or being at different stages of disease [31, 36, 37]. However, the predictive value of the findings obtained in these studies is difficult to interpret, mainly because the results may have been affected by the clinical manifestations of the patients and the therapeutic procedures they were going through. A clearer view of the prognostic value of CCL5 serum levels in breast cancer patients would necessitate standardization of the studies performed in this respect. Specifically, it is important to determine the plasma levels of the chemokine prior to any treatment of the patients, since CCL5 circulating levels may reflect immune functions that come into effect following the exposure of patients to various immunization procedures or to different therapeutic regimens.

As a potential pro-malignancy factor in breast cancer, CCL5 activities necessitate the expression of its corresponding receptors by potential target cells, therefore a number of studies have analyzed the associations between breast malignancy and the CCR5 receptor for CCL5. The discovery of the CCR5Δ32 polymorphism that leads to a mutated dysfunctional CCR5 [50] has enabled researchers to more specifically analyze the involvement of CCR5 in breast cancer. The research by Manes et al. suggested that CCR5 has a protective role in breast cancer in a mechanism mediated by p53, and has shown that individuals bearing a nonfunctional CCR5Δ32 had a shorter disease-free survival than patients having wild-type CCR5 [51]. However, it is important to note that the results of other studies that have looked at the association of the CCR5Δ32 mutation with breast cancer progression have not seen any associations between the two parameters [52–54].

Taken together, the analyses based on the CCR5Δ32 mutation have not led to definite conclusions on the roles played by CCR5 in breast cancer. In contrast, other approaches strongly supported a tumor-promoting function for CCR5 in this disease. The genetic analysis provided in the study by Bieche et al. [33] revealed significant upregulation of CCR5 expression in IBC patients, as compared to non-IBC patients, suggesting that CCR5 is involved in a more aggressive type of disease. Also, the use of the met-CCL5 antagonist of CCR5/CCR1 and of siRNA to CCR5, has led to significant inhibition of breast malignancy in animal model systems [39, 48], suggesting that CCR5 has protumorigenic effects in this disease.

Therefore, direct analyses of CCR5 indicate that it supports breast malignancy, but thus far this possibility was not backed up by studies of the CCR5Δ32 polymorphism. It is possible that efforts to more definitely decipher the roles of CCR5 in this disease are hampered by the fact that this receptor acts in parallel to CCR1 and CCR3, and is activated by other ligands in addition to CCL5. To date, it is not known to which degree each of the three receptors mediates the activities of CCL5 in breast cancer, and in what manner. The possibility exists that it is the equilibrium between the three receptors and their corresponding chemokine ligands that eventually dictates the malignancy and metastatic cascades in breast cancer.

The identification of CCL5 association with advanced breast cancer or with progression raised the question whether the chemokine is merely correlated with advanced disease course, or rather, does it play an active role in disease development and progression. In this respect, several studies performed in murine model systems strongly supported a causative role for the CCL5/CCR5 axis in breast malignancy. Downregulation of CCL5 expression by antisense has led to reduced tumor growth of 4T1 murine mammary tumor cells, and to a significant inhibition of liver and brain metastasis [46, 47]. Although contradictory findings were later provided by the same group [55], other studies further supported the direct involvement of CCL5 in breast malignancy. The recent study by Weinberg's group has shown that inhibition of CCL5 by neutralizing antibodies or of CCR5 expression by siRNA, impaired the tumor-supporting roles that were mediated by a CCL5–CCR5 loop [39]. This investigation also showed that over-expression of CCL5 in breast tumor cells led to increased lung metastasis [39]. Moreover, the study by Robinson et al. indicated that inhibition of CCL5 activities by the met-CCL5 antagonist of CCR5 and CCR1 induced a significant reduction in tumor volume and weight, resulting from transplantation with 410.4 murine mammary carcinoma cells [48].

The causative roles attributed to CCL5 in breast cancer motivated the search for better identification of its modes of action in this disease. First, it is possible that the chemokine acts directly on the cancer cells to promote their ability to exert promalignancy properties. Such an activity of the chemokine necessitates the expression of the corresponding receptors for CCL5 by the tumor cells. Indeed, CCL5 was found to bind to breast tumor cells, and CCR5 and CCR1 receptors were detected in breast tumor cells in culture and/or in biopsies of breast cancer patients ([39–41, 43, 46, 56–58] and A. Ben-Baruch et al., unpublished results).

In line with the expression of CCL5 receptors by breast tumor cells, the chemokine was found to promote tumor cell motility and invasion, but apparently not proliferation [39, 43, 56, 57]. Actually, CCL5 was found to be involved in the regulation of breast tumor cell migration and invasion at several levels. Recent findings indicated that insulin-like growth factor (IGF)-I induced the migration of breast tumor cells, in a mechanism necessitating transactivation of CCR5 via transcriptional upregulation and secretion of CCL5 [43]. Additional research was performed on the regulation of breast tumor cell migration by c-Myc, using the human breast cancer lines MCF-7 and MDA-MB-231. This study has provided evidence for an intricate regulation by c-MYC, and showed that in MCF-7 cells its depletion induced upregulation of CCL5 expression, leading to increased migration of the MCF-7 cells [44]. Further proof of the involvement of CCL5 in breast tumor cell invasion was provided recently by the study of Weinberg and his colleagues, showing that mesenchymal stem cells release the chemokine in response to stimulation by breast tumor cells, and that the chemokine in turn induces tumor cell migration and promotes invasion and metastasis [39].

Together, these findings indicate that CCL5 promotes tumor cell motility and invasion, leading to elevated metastatic potential. Such an activity of the chemokine is complemented by its ability to upregulate the release of matrix metalloproteinase (MMP) 9 by breast tumor cells [40], and indeed high CCL5 expression was associated with increased expression of extracellular matrix-degrading enzymes [46, 47]. In addition, it was recently proposed that CCL5 may support metastasis by acting on cells of the tumor microenvironment and promoting angiogenesis [40, 41, 59, 60], by facilitating the metastatic spread of tumor cells.

Further related to the promalignancy activities of CCL5 on cells of the tumor microenvironment, the chemokine supports breast malignancy by changing the equilibrium between leukocyte infiltrates in breast tumors, leading to dominance of cells with tumor-promoting activities at the tumor site. The major hematopoietic infiltrates residing in breast tumors are tumor-associated macrophages (TAM), having deleterious activities at the tumor site. These cells were significantly associated with breast cancer progression and were found to support breast malignancy via their ability to express a large variety of tumor-promoting factors [1, 2, 5, 6, 61–67]. The elevated presence of TAM in breast tumors is the result of monocyte migration from the circulation into the tumor, where the monocytes then differentiate into TAM. Strong evidence, opposed by only one study, supports the ability of CCL5 to promote the attraction of such monocytes and of myeloid cells to breast tumor sites [39, 40, 45, 47, 48]. Furthermore, the chemokine was shown to upregulate the release of tumor-supporting factors in monocytes, such as MMP and angiogenic factors [40, 41, 68–70], raising the possibility that CCL5 stimulates the secretion of promalignancy mediators by TAM.

The ability of CCL5 to promote monocyte migration to breast tumors is complemented by its roles in reducing the infiltration and activation of potential antitumor T cells. The model system of CCL5-expressing 4T1 mammary tumors has shown that expression of the chemokine is associated with desensitization of T-cell migration, with increased tumor growth, with lower levels of CD3-expressing infiltrating lymphocytes, and with reduced T-cell immune activities [42, 47]. Moreover, CCL5 was found to induce MMP9 expression in splenic T cells [47], representing another mechanism by which it may contribute to breast malignancy via modification of hematopoietic cells at the tumor microenvironment.

Overall, the above studies indicate that CCL5 changes the balance between infiltrating hematopoietic cells in breast tumors, shifting the equilibrium in favor of tumor-promoting TAM and against potentially protective T cells. However, it should be noted that under specific conditions the rejection of mammary tumors was accompanied by CCL5 expression, often associated with increased infiltration of different leukocyte populations to the tumors, primarily T cells [71–75]. It is therefore possible that at certain stages of the malignant process, CCL5 could be exploited by the host for defense against the developing tumor.

Evidence for a protective role for CCL5 in breast cancer stems from studies in animal model systems, and the relevance of these findings to potential antitumor activities of CCL5 in breast cancer patients is not substantiated as yet. It could be that at initial stages of disease, CCL5 has the potential to elicit T-cell immune activities, and also to recruit monocytes with antitumor functions. However, when the expression of the chemokine is elevated, it is skewed to a promalignancy factor that promotes tumor-supporting activities in the tumor cells and in cells of the tumor microenvironment. What is it then that stimulates the release of the chemokine by the tumor cells? T cells and monocytes that have been recruited to the tumor site at initial stages of the process may secrete IFNγ and TNFα, leading to induction of CCL5 by the tumor cells. Eventually, the increased secretion of CCL5 by the tumor cells may skew the tumor microenvironment toward a promalignancy phenotype, joined by direct tumor-promoting activities of the chemokine on the tumor cells.

To conclude, based on many findings – derived from studies done in breast cancer patients, in animal model systems, and in in vitro systems – it is believed that CCL5 and CCR5 have been diverted into tumor-supporting properties that play key and causative roles in breast cancer development and progression. Although many additional aspects related to the activities of CCL5/CCR5 pair in breast cancer should be clarified, based on the currently available information we suggest that this axis is an appropriate and important therapeutic target in breast cancer.

Melanoma

The studies on chemokines and their receptors provided evidence that several members of this superfamily support growth of melanoma cells (primarily CXCL8 and CXCL1-3) and promote organ-specific metastasis (CXCR4, CCR7, and CCR10) [7, 76]. Side by side with these research directions, the functions of tumor-infiltrating lymphocytes (TILs) with antimalignancy effects in melanoma were described [77–80]. The findings on TIL raised the possibility that specific chemokines may inhibit melanoma progression by recruiting T cells to the tumor site, thus promoting immune surveillance in melanoma. Therefore, a search has begun on the possible roles played by definite chemokines in attracting T cells to melanomas. These studies addressed the involvement of the CCL5/CCR5 axis in this disease, and its association with immune activities against melanoma cells.

First, the different investigations showed that CCL5 was expressed by melanoma cells, and CCR5 expression was detected in primary melanomas and melanoma cutaneous metastasis [81–85]. Focusing on CCL5, its expression at the mRNA and/or protein levels was detected in several, but not all, melanoma cell lines and in fine needle aspirates of melanoma cells from patients [81–84]. CCL5 expression was higher in melanomas than in normal melanocytes, and was associated with a higher malignancy state and increased tumor formation [81, 82], therefore suggesting elevated activities of the CCL5/CCR5 axis in more advanced stages of disease.

These findings on the potential promalignancy roles of CCL5 in melanoma raised concerns regarding the actual ability of this chemokine to induce antitumor cell activities in melanoma. While the study by Dobrzanski et al. suggested a correlation between CCL5 expression and increased numbers of host-derived immune cells in lung metastasis in a melanoma model [86], other studies have clearly implicated a tumor-promoting role for CCR5, and a defective function of CCR5-expressing hematopoietic cells in melanoma [87–89]. In addition to a lower malignancy phenotype observed in CCR5-/- mice [88, 89], the study by Mellado et al. has shown that CCR5 plays a key role in induction of apoptotic death in human melanoma-derived TIL, in a CCL5-dependent manner [87]. The findings also indicated that CXCL12 released by melanoma cells induced the expression of CCL5 by infiltrating lymphocytes, which in turn activated a death program in TIL [87]. This activity was not limited only to CCL5 and was upregulated also by CCL3 and CCL4, acting through CCR5 to induce cyto-chrome c release into the cytosol, and leading to activation of caspase-9 and caspase-3.

The above study suggested a potential mechanism through which mela-noma cells can induce immune escape from potential antitumor activities of T cells, in a process mediated via TIL-expressed CCR5. Two additional studies raised the possibility that CCR5 provides support to the developing tumor cells: using a murine B16 melanoma system, Serody and colleagues found that the lack of CCR5 in the host mouse gave rise to delayed melanoma growth and lung metastases. The two studies have carefully analyzed the mechanisms by which the lack of CCR5 may endow protection to the host against melanoma growth, suggesting a complex array of events including the involvement of hematopoietic and stroma cells in CCR5-mediated increase in tumor growth and metastasis [88–90].

The above studies suggest an association between CCR5 and increased tumor growth in melanoma, possibly through an imbalance in immune activ-ities. However, when the presence of the CCR5Δ32 polymorphism was con-sidered, it has led to opposing findings: while the study by Rodero et al. did not find an association between this polymorphism and melanoma susceptibility and progression [91], another investigation has shown in stage IV melanoma patients a significant correlation of the CCR5Δ32 mutation with decreased survival following immunotherapy [92].

Taken together, while the studies on CCL5 show a significant association between the chemokine and progressed melanoma, it is not clear what are the exact roles of CCR5 in this process, and whether impaired activities of CCR5-expressing immune cells play a role in this disease. Further contributing to the enigma in this respect are studies done on dendritic cells (DC) in melanoma. The findings presented in the study by Ng-Cashin et al. showed that the absence of CCR5 expression in the host has led to decrease in early tumor growth, and that DC-based vaccination in CCR5-/- mice resulted in complete regression [88]. Based on the observations made in this study, it was suggested that blocking the activity of CCR5 in the host should be considered as a strategy to enhance the activities of DC vaccines in melanoma. However, other studies have revealed inconsistencies with regard to the roles played by the CCL5/CCR5 axis in DC-mediated immune surveillance. It was shown that melanoma cells led to increased E-cadherin expression in DC, therefore preventing their migration, in a process mediated by a soluble factor, although probably not CCL5 [93]. Adding further to the ambiguity regarding CCR5 effects on DC activities in melanoma, it was found that DC that have phagocytosed apoptotic/necrotic melanoma cells had enhanced antitumor activity that was associated with upregulation of CCL3 and CCL4 [94].

Overall, when all the findings on CCL5/CCR5 and their associated members in melanoma are taken together, the majority of studies suggests that CCL5 expression is associated with melanoma progression. Additional investigations provide evidence of a CCL5/CCR5-mediated imbalance in T cell and DC activities that may support such a process. However, there are many unresolved issues with respect to the exact roles of this axis in regulation of T cell and DC activities, raising the need for extensive research on the implications of CCL5 and CCR5 in melanoma.

Gastric Cancer

The studies that have analyzed the expression of CCL5 in gastric cancer focused mainly on its potential roles and predictive value in metastasis. The possibility that CCL5 could serve as a predictor of metastasis was based on a study analyzing CCL5 circulating levels in 109 gastric cancer patients, prior to anti-cancer treatment. This study has shown that the plasma levels of the chemokine were significantly higher in patients than in healthy controls, and in stage IV patients as compared to patients diagnosed in stages I or II–III of disease [95].

The possibility that increased CCL5 levels are indicative of metastasis was thereafter supported by a study analyzing the mRNA expression of the chemokine in human gastric cancer cell lines that were selected for a high-metastatic potential. Comparison of these cell lines to their low-metastatic parental variants indicated that the cells that have acquired a metastatic potential had an upregulated CCL5 gene expression [96]. Also, the transcripts of CCL5 were elevated in a gastric cancer model system following infection by *Helicobacter pylori*, and were reduced by administration of anti-inflammatory drugs [97]. This latter inhibition agreed with the characterization of this chemokine as an inflammatory factor, and emphasized the potential roles played by inflammatory mediators in this disease.

The above studies suggested a tumor-promoting role of CCL5 in gastric cancer. This possibility was supported by a study analyzing the effects of supernatants derived from low- and high-metastatic gastric cancer cell lines on the activities of peripheral blood mononuclear cells (PBMC). The study showed that exposure of the PBMC to supernatants of highly metastatic gastric cancer cell lines gave rise to elevated CCL5 expression by the PBMC, as compared to PBMC stimulated by supernatants of low-metastatic cells. In turn, tumor cells cocultured with PBMC had higher invasion properties than noncocultured cells, and this process was highly inhibited by antibodies to CCL5. These results suggest that tumor-cell cooperation with PBMC, possibly through CCL5 potentiates invasion of the tumor cells [98].

However, as was the case in other malignancies, the roles of leukocytes in gastric cancer were not fully deciphered to date. The study of patients that underwent gastrectomy due to gastric cancer revealed infiltration of CD8+ T cells that contained CCL5+ cytoplasmic granules similar to inflammatory lesions of chronic gastritis. The findings of this research suggested a self-recruiting mechanism involving CCR5 and CCL5 for tissue accumulation of T cells, and a role for the CCL5-enriched T cells in protection against the tumor cells [99]. Of note, since there was no correlation between CCR5+ cells and cancer stage in this study, this possibility has to be fully substantiated.

The implications of this latter study are not clear as yet, but they should be viewed in the context of the other studies, suggesting a promalignancy role of the CCL5/CCR5 axis in gastric cancer. Obviously, there is a need to continue the research on this pair, and to more clearly elucidate the effects of CCL5 on different target cells, including the tumor cells and immune cells in gastric cancer.

Ovarian Cancer

The studies addressing the CCL5/CCR5 axis in ovarian carcinoma have analyzed the expression of the chemokine and of its receptor by the tumor cells and by infiltrating leukocytes. CCL5 expression was detected in malignant ovarian biopsies, but also in normal biopsies, with minimal expression in ovarian cancer cell lines [100–103]. The cell type expressing CCL5 in the biopsies was not fully determined, but it was suggested that infiltrating leukocytes constitute the major origin of the chemokine in ovarian tumors [102].

Evidence supporting an association between CCL5 and ovarian carcinoma progression was provided by a study analyzing the levels of the chemokine in plasma of patients at different stages of disease. This study has shown that CCL5 protein levels were higher in ovarian cancer patients than in patients diagnosed with benign ovarian cysts, and elevated in stages III–IV of ovarian cancer compared to stages I–II [104]. This study suggested that pre-operative CCL5 levels could be useful for detection of malignant ovarian tumors.

In addition to studies done on ovarian cancer biopsies and serum, mRNA and/or protein level analyses identified the expression of CCL5 in ascitic fluids of ovarian carcinoma patients, and showed that CCL5 expression was significantly associated with the expression of the other two ligands of CCR5, CCL3, and CCL4 [105]. Also, the expression of CCL5 was higher in ascites with high prevalence of CD3+ cells, and its expression was correlated with CD8+ T cells [102, 105].

These investigations suggested that CCL5 expression may be indicative of immune activities in breast cancer patients. As such, it was expected that the expression of CCL5 receptors by hematopoietic cells would provide insights into the roles of this chemokine in ovarian cancer. Along these lines, the expression of CCR5 and CCR1 was detected in cells from ovarian ascites, mainly by leukocytes. CCR1 was expressed by the majority of CD8+ T cells, but more CD4+ than CD8+ T cells expressed CCR5 [105]. Also, CCR5 expression was detected on monocytes in pleural effusions; however, only rare expression of CCR5 was detected in the tumor cells [105, 106].

The expression of CCL5 receptors by leukocytes in ovarian cancer raises questions on the roles played by such cells in disease course. In a study performed in vivo with the OV-HM ovarian carcinoma cell line, tumor rejection was induced by interleukin-12 (IL-12), in a process mediated by CCR5. This study has shown that following IL-12 treatment, CCR5 mRNA was elevated in splenic T cells, and that the levels of its CCL3 and CCL4 ligands were elevated in the tumor mass [107]. Also, T-cell infiltrates in this model expressed CCR5, and using the CCR5 antagonist TAK-779 in tumor-bearing mice prevented IL-12-induced tumor regression, as well as T-cell migration [107]. Therefore, this study suggests a protective role for CCR5+ lymphocytes in ovarian cancer. In contrast to the above study, implying that CCR5+ lymphocytes have anti-tumorigenic roles in ovarian cancer, CCL5 was suggested to be responsible for elevated presence of deleterious TAM in ovarian tumors [108].

When all the findings on CCL5 and CCR5 in ovarian cancer are considered together, it is as yet too early to make any definite conclusion on the roles they play in this disease. It is possible that CCL5 acts differently on various leukocyte subpopulations, having opposing effects on activities exerted by T cells and macrophages. Also, it is not clear whether the chemokine directly affects the tumor cells themselves, or other host cells at the tumor microenvironment in ovarian cancer. Therefore, at present the roles played by this chemokine and its receptors in ovarian cancer are far from being resolved, and many additional aspects should be studied in this disease.

Conclusions

The investigation of the roles played by CCL5 and CCR5 in tumor development and metastasis is only beginning. While promalignancy effects for the CCL5/CCR5 and their associated members are strongly implicated in MM and breast cancer, their contribution to other malignancies is only starting to be unraveled. Initial steps were taken in melanoma, gastric cancer, and ovarian carcinoma, providing preliminary evidence for the roles played by the CCL5/CCR5 axis in these diseases. In other cancer types, the findings are mainly descriptive, providing only hints of the possible activities of CCL5 and CCR5 in disease progression (e.g., in hepatocellular carcinoma [109–116]).

The findings described in this chapter emphasize the need for further research on the roles played by the CCL5/CCR5 pair in malignancy. CCL5, as well as other ligands of CCR5, are chemoattractants to immune/inflammatory cells, and thus may have the potential to promote antitumor activities under specific circumstances. However, the studies that were performed thus far on MM and breast cancer suggest that in specific malignancies the promalignancy effects of the CCL5/CCR5 axis dominate such potential beneficial effects, eventually leading to tumor development and/or progression.

It is therefore obligatory to pinpoint with better accuracy the roles of this pair in each specific malignancy, to identify the exact conditions in which they exert protumorigenic activities, and the circumstances in which they could be exploited in benefit of the host. However, reaching a clear-cut conclusion on the roles of CCL5 and CCR5 in cancer is hampered by the promiscuity and redundancy that characterize them. This is mainly so because the activities of other ligands of CCR5 (CCL3 and CCL4) and of additional CCL5 receptors (CCR1 and CCR3) may come into effect and dictate the final impact of these components in malignancy.

The characteristics of all factors involved in the activities of CCL5/CCR5 should be also considered when therapeutics are designed. Obviously, if there are specific malignancies in which CCL5 and CCR5 prominently support tumor progression, it would be reasonable to search for modalities that reduce their activities and/or expression. Choosing the CCL5/CCR5 axis as a therapeutic target in cancer fits well with laborious efforts currently taken in order to block HIV infectivity via CCR5, as well as to reduce inflammatory diseases. It is therefore possible that drugs which are being designed for such purposes would prove effective also in specific malignancies in which CCL5 acts through CCR5 to support cancerous processes.

However, the design of CCL5/CCR5 inhibitors should be considered in the framework of the promiscuity and redundancy of the receptor and of the ligand. More specifically, the question is whether the design of drugs that are highly specific only for this pair is advantageous over modalities that impair the binding and activities of all high-affinity CCR5 ligands, and/or the other receptors for CCL5. This depends very much on the equilibrium between all these components in specific malignancies, as well as in normal hematopoietic processes.

Furthermore, one has to take into account the fact that the CCL5/CCR5 axis acts in conjunction with other chemokines to affect the malignancy phenotype (e.g., the CXCL12/CXCR4 pair), exemplifying the multifactorial nature of malignancies and the need to target several mediators simultaneously. Also, in considering CCL5 and CCR5 as therapeutic targets, we should consider the effects of anti-CCL5/CCR5 treatments on the immune integrity of the host. The optimal therapeutic modalities would have to accommodate two opposing demands: the need to inhibit the detrimental involvement of CCL5 and CCR5 in specific malignant diseases, but protect their potentially beneficial activities in immunity, including in cancer.

Overall, our current knowledge leads us to suggest the CCL5/CCR5 axis as a potential therapeutic target in several cancer diseases. However, bringing this proposal into practical application requires further in depth research, to insure that such treatments are supported by the appropriate rationale.

Acknowledgments The relevant research to this paper, which is performed in the authors' laboratory, is supported by The Israel Academy of Sciences and Humanities; The Israel Cancer Association; The Israel Ministry of Health; The Ela Kodesz Institute for Research on Cancer Development and Prevention; The Federico Foundation. The authors thank the members of the laboratory and collaborators who have contributed to the studies on chemokines in malignancy and in inflammation.

References

1. Ben-Baruch, A. 2006. The multifaceted roles of chemokines in malignancy. *Cancer Metastasis Rev* 25:357.
2. Conti, I., and B. J. Rollins. 2004. CCL2 (monocyte chemoattractant protein-1) and cancer. *Semin Cancer Biol* 14:149.
3. Zlotnik, A. 2006. Involvement of chemokine receptors in organ-specific metastasis. *Contrib Microbiol* 13:191.
4. Strieter, R. M., M. D. Burdick, J. Mestas, B. Gomperts, M. P. Keane, and J. A. Belperio. 2006. Cancer CXC chemokine networks and tumour angiogenesis. *Eur J Cancer* 42:768.
5. Ben-Baruch, A. 2006. *Pro-malignancy and putative anti-malignancy chemokines in the regulation of breast cancer progression.* Nova Science Publishers.
6. Ben-Baruch, A. 2006. Inflammation-associated immune suppression in cancer: the roles played by cytokines, chemokines and additional mediators. *Semin Cancer Biol* 16:38.
7. Ben-Baruch, A. 2008. Organ selectivity in metastasis: regulation by chemokines and their receptors. *Clin Exp Metastasis* 25:345.
8. Wong, M. M., and E. N. Fish. 2003. Chemokines: attractive mediators of the immune response. *Semin Immunol* 15:5.
9. Mueller, A., and P. G. Strange. 2004. The chemokine receptor, CCR5. *Int J Biochem Cell Biol* 36:35.
10. Luther, S. A., and J. G. Cyster. 2001. Chemokines as regulators of T cell differentiation. *Nat Immunol* 2:102.
11. Sallusto, F., C. R. Mackay, and A. Lanzavecchia. 2000. The role of chemokine receptors in primary, effector, and memory immune responses. *Annu Rev Immunol* 18:593.
12. Mackay, C. R., and F. Sallusto. 2006. A new role for CCR5 in innate immunity–binding to bacterial heat shock protein 70. *Eur J Immunol* 36:2293.
13. Murphy, P. M., M. Baggiolini, I. F. Charo, C. A. Hebert, R. Horuk, K. Matsushima, L. H. Miller, J. J. Oppenheim, and C. A. Power. 2000. International union of pharmacology. XXII. Nomenclature for chemokine receptors. *Pharmacol Rev* 52:145.
14. Bacon, K., M. Baggiolini, H. Broxmeyer, R. Horuk, I. Lindley, A. Mantovani, K. Maysushima, P. Murphy, H. Nomiyama, J. Oppenheim, A. Rot, T. Schall, M. Tsang, R. Thorpe, J. Van Damme, M. Wadhwa, O. Yoshie, A. Zlotnik, and K. Zoon. 2002. Chemokine/chemokine receptor nomenclature. *J Interferon Cytokine Res* 22:1067.
15. Devalaraja, M. N., and A. Richmond. 1999. Multiple chemotactic factors: fine control or redundancy? *Trends Pharmacol Sci* 20:151.
16. Mantovani, A. 1999. The chemokine system: redundancy for robust outputs. *Immunol Today* 20:254.
17. Abe, M., K. Hiura, J. Wilde, K. Moriyama, T. Hashimoto, S. Ozaki, S. Wakatsuki, M. Kosaka, S. Kido, D. Inoue, and T. Matsumoto. 2002. Role for macrophage inflammatory protein (MIP)-1alpha and MIP-1beta in the development of osteolytic lesions in multiple myeloma. *Blood* 100:2195.

18. Oba, Y., J. W. Lee, L. A. Ehrlich, H. Y. Chung, D. F. Jelinek, N. S. Callander, R. Horuk, S. J. Choi, and G. D. Roodman. 2005. MIP-1alpha utilizes both CCR1 and CCR5 to induce osteoclast formation and increase adhesion of myeloma cells to marrow stromal cells. *Exp Hematol* 33:272.

19. Menu, E., E. De Leenheer, H. De Raeve, L. Coulton, T. Imanishi, K. Miyashita, E. Van Valckenborgh, I. Van Riet, B. Van Camp, R. Horuk, P. Croucher, and K. Vanderkerken. 2006. Role of CCR1 and CCR5 in homing and growth of multiple myeloma and in the development of osteolytic lesions: a study in the 5TMM model. *Clin Exp Metastasis* 23:291.

20. Choi, S. J., J. C. Cruz, F. Craig, H. Chung, R. D. Devlin, G. D. Roodman, and M. Alsina. 2000. Macrophage inflammatory protein 1-alpha is a potential osteoclast stimulatory factor in multiple myeloma. *Blood* 96:671.

21. Lentzsch, S., M. Gries, M. Janz, R. Bargou, B. Dorken, and M. Y. Mapara. 2003. Macrophage inflammatory protein 1-alpha (MIP-1 alpha) triggers migration and signaling cascades mediating survival and proliferation in multiple myeloma (MM) cells. *Blood* 101:3568.

22. Hashimoto, T., M. Abe, T. Oshima, H. Shibata, S. Ozaki, D. Inoue, and T. Matsumoto. 2004. Ability of myeloma cells to secrete macrophage inflammatory protein (MIP)-1alpha and MIP-1beta correlates with lytic bone lesions in patients with multiple myeloma. *Br J Haematol* 125:38.

23. Terpos, E., M. Politou, R. Szydlo, J. M. Goldman, J. F. Apperley, and A. Rahemtulla. 2003. Serum levels of macrophage inflammatory protein-1 alpha (MIP-1alpha) correlate with the extent of bone disease and survival in patients with multiple myeloma. *Br J Haematol* 123:106.

24. Terpos, E., M. Politou, N. Viniou, and A. Rahemtulla. 2005. Significance of macrophage inflammatory protein-1 alpha (MIP-1alpha) in multiple myeloma. *Leuk Lymphoma* 46:1699.

25. Choi, S. J., Y. Oba, Y. Gazitt, M. Alsina, J. Cruz, J. Anderson, and G. D. Roodman. 2001. Antisense inhibition of macrophage inflammatory protein 1-alpha blocks bone destruction in a model of myeloma bone disease. *J Clin Invest* 108:1833.

26. Lentzsch, S., M. Chatterjee, M. Gries, K. Bommert, H. Gollasch, B. Dorken, and R. C. Bargou. 2004. PI3-K/AKT/FKHR and MAPK signaling cascades are redundantly stimulated by a variety of cytokines and contribute independently to proliferation and survival of multiple myeloma cells. *Leukemia* 18:1883.

27. Han, J. H., S. J. Choi, N. Kurihara, M. Koide, Y. Oba, and G. D. Roodman. 2001. Macrophage inflammatory protein-1alpha is an osteoclastogenic factor in myeloma that is independent of receptor activator of nuclear factor kappaB ligand. *Blood* 97:3349.

28. Trentin, L., M. Miorin, M. Facco, I. Baesso, S. Carraro, A. Cabrelle, N. Maschio, M. Bortoli, G. Binotto, F. Piazza, F. Adami, R. Zambello, C. Agostini, and G. Semenzato. 2007. Multiple myeloma plasma cells show different chemokine receptor profiles at sites of disease activity. *Br J Haematol* 138:594.

29. Moller, C., T. Stromberg, M. Juremalm, K. Nilsson, and G. Nilsson. 2003. Expression and function of chemokine receptors in human multiple myeloma. *Leukemia* 17:203.

30. Luboshits, G., S. Shina, O. Kaplan, S. Engelberg, D. Nass, B. Lifshitz-Mercer, S. Chaitchik, I. Keydar, and A. Ben-Baruch. 1999. Elevated expression of the CC chemokine regulated on activation, normal T cell expressed and secreted (RANTES) in advanced breast carcinoma. *Cancer Res* 59:4681.

31. Niwa, Y., H. Akamatsu, H. Niwa, H. Sumi, Y. Ozaki, and A. Abe. 2001. Correlation of tissue and plasma RANTES levels with disease course in patients with breast or cervical cancer. *Clin Cancer Res* 7:285.

32. Yaal-Hahoshen, N., S. Shina, L. Leider-Trejo, I. Barnea, E. L. Shabtai, E. Azenshtein, I. Greenberg, I. Keydar, and A. Ben-Baruch. 2006. The chemokine CCL5 as a potential prognostic factor predicting disease progression in stage II breast cancer patients. *Clin Cancer Res* 12:4474.

33. Bieche, I., F. Lerebours, S. Tozlu, M. Espie, M. Marty, and R. Lidereau. 2004. Molecular profiling of inflammatory breast cancer: identification of a poor-prognosis gene expression signature. *Clin Cancer Res* 10:6789.

34. Tedla, N., P. Palladinetti, D. Wakefield, and A. Lloyd. 1999. Abundant expression of chemokines in malignant and infective human lymphadenopathies. *Cytokine* 11:531.
35. Celis, J. E., P. Gromov, T. Cabezon, J. M. Moreira, N. Ambartsumian, K. Sandelin, F. Rank, and I. Gromova. 2004. Proteomic characterization of the interstitial fluid perfusing the breast tumor microenvironment: a novel resource for biomarker and therapeutic target discovery. *Mol Cell Proteomics* 3:327.
36. Dehqanzada, Z. A., C. E. Storrer, M. T. Hueman, R. J. Foley, K. A. Harris, Y. H. Jama, C. D. Shriver, S. Ponniah, and G. E. Peoples. 2007. Assessing serum cytokine profiles in breast cancer patients receiving a HER2/neu vaccine using Luminex technology. *Oncol Rep* 17:687.
37. Eissa, S. A., S. A. Zaki, S. M. El-Maghraby, and D. Y. Kadry. 2005. Importance of serum IL-18 and RANTES as markers for breast carcinoma progression. *J Egypt Natl Canc Inst* 17:51.
38. Wigler, N., S. Shina, O. Kaplan, G. Luboshits, S. Chaitchik, I. Keydar, and A. Ben-Baruch. 2002. Breast carcinoma: a report on the potential usage of the CC chemokine RANTES as a marker for a progressive disease. *Isr Med Assoc J* 4:940.
39. Karnoub, A. E., A. B. Dash, A. P. Vo, A. Sullivan, M. W. Brooks, G. W. Bell, A. L. Richardson, K. Polyak, R. Tubo, and R. A. Weinberg. 2007. Mesenchymal stem cells within tumour stroma promote breast cancer metastasis. *Nature* 449:557.
40. Azenshtein, E., G. Luboshits, S. Shina, E. Neumark, D. Shahbazian, M. Weil, N. Wigler, I. Keydar, and A. Ben-Baruch. 2002. The CC chemokine RANTES in breast carcinoma progression: regulation of expression and potential mechanisms of promalignant activity. *Cancer Res* 62:1093.
41. Azenshtein, E., T. Meshel, S. Shina, N. Barak, I. Keydar, and A. Ben-Baruch. 2005. The angiogenic factors CXCL8 and VEGF in breast cancer: regulation by an array of pro-malignancy factors. *Cancer Lett* 217:73.
42. Kurt, R. A., A. Baher, K. P. Wisner, S. Tackitt, and W. J. Urba. 2001. Chemokine receptor desensitization in tumor-bearing mice. *Cell Immunol* 207:81.
43. Mira, E., R. A. Lacalle, M. A. Gonzalez, C. Gomez-Mouton, J. L. Abad, A. Bernad, A. C. Martinez, and S. Manes. 2001. A role for chemokine receptor transactivation in growth factor signaling. *EMBO Rep* 2:151.
44. Cappellen, D., T. Schlange, M. Bauer, F. Maurer, and N. E. Hynes. 2007. Novel c-MYC target genes mediate differential effects on cell proliferation and migration. *EMBO Rep* 8:70.
45. Dupre, S. A., D. Redelman, and K. W. Hunter, Jr. 2007. The mouse mammary carcinoma 4T1: characterization of the cellular landscape of primary tumours and metastatic tumour foci. *Int J Exp Pathol* 88:351.
46. Stormes, K. A., C. A. Lemken, J. V. Lepre, M. N. Marinucci, and R. A. Kurt. 2005. Inhibition of metastasis by inhibition of tumor-derived CCL5. *Breast Cancer Res Treat* 89:209.
47. Adler, E. P., C. A. Lemken, N. S. Katchen, and R. A. Kurt. 2003. A dual role for tumor-derived chemokine RANTES (CCL5). *Immunol Lett* 90:187.
48. Robinson, S. C., K. A. Scott, J. L. Wilson, R. G. Thompson, A. E. Proudfoot, and F. R. Balkwill. 2003. A chemokine receptor antagonist inhibits experimental breast tumor growth. *Cancer Res* 63:8360.
49. Ali, S., J. Kaur, and K. D. Patel. 2000. Intercellular cell adhesion molecule-1, vascular cell adhesion molecule-1, and regulated on activation normal T cell expressed and secreted are expressed by human breast carcinoma cells and support eosinophil adhesion and activation. *Am J Pathol* 157:313.
50. de Silva, E., and M. P. Stumpf. 2004. HIV and the CCR5-Delta32 resistance allele. *FEMS Microbiol Lett* 241:1.
51. Manes, S., E. Mira, R. Colomer, S. Montero, L. M. Real, C. Gomez-Mouton, S. Jimenez-Baranda, A. Garzon, R. A. Lacalle, K. Harshman, A. Ruiz, and A. C. Martinez. 2003. CCR5 expression influences the progression of human breast cancer in a p53-dependent manner. *J Exp Med* 198:1381.

52. Degerli, N., E. Yilmaz, and F. Bardakci. 2005. The Delta32 allele distribution of the CCR5 gene and its relationship with certain cancers in a Turkish population. *Clin Biochem* 38:248.
53. Ghilardi, G., M. L. Biondi, A. La Torre, L. Battaglioli, and R. Scorza. 2005. Breast cancer progression and host polymorphisms in the chemokine system: role of the macrophage chemoattractant protein-1 (MCP-1) -2518 G allele. *Clin Chem* 51:452.
54. Zafiropoulos, A., N. Crikas, A. M. Passam, and D. A. Spandidos. 2004. Significant involvement of CCR2-64I and CXCL12-3a in the development of sporadic breast cancer. *J Med Genet* 41: e59.
55. Jayasinghe, M. M., J.M. Golden, P. Nair, C. M. O'Donnell, M. T. Werner, and R. A. Kurt. 2008. Tumor-derived CCL5 does not contribute to breast cancer progression. *Breast Cancer Res Treat* 111:511.
56. Prest, S. J., R. C. Rees, C. Murdoch, J. F. Marshall, P. A. Cooper, M. Bibby, G. Li, and S. A. Ali. 1999. Chemokines induce the cellular migration of MCF-7 human breast carcinoma cells: subpopulations of tumour cells display positive and negative chemotaxis and differential in vivo growth potentials. *Clin Exp Metastasis* 17:389.
57. Youngs, S. J., S. A. Ali, D. D. Taub, and R. C. Rees. 1997. Chemokines induce migrational responses in human breast carcinoma cell lines. *Int J Cancer* 71:257.
58. Aronica, S. M., P. Fanti, K. Kaminskaya, K. Gibbs, L. Raiber, M. Nazareth, R. Bucelli, M. Mineo, K. Grzybek, M. Kumin, K. Poppenberg, C. Schwach, and K. Janis. 2004. Estrogen disrupts chemokine-mediated chemokine release from mammary cells: implications for the interplay between estrogen and IP-10 in the regulation of mammary tumor formation. *Breast Cancer Res Treat* 84:235.
59. Khodarev, N. N., J. Yu, E. Labay, T. Darga, C. K. Brown, H. J. Mauceri, R. Yassari, N. Gupta, and R. R. Weichselbaum. 2003. Tumour-endothelium interactions in co-culture: coordinated changes of gene expression profiles and phenotypic properties of endothelial cells. *J Cell Sci* 116:1013.
60. Sun, X. T., M. Y. Zhang, C. Shu, Q. Li, X. G. Yan, N. Cheng, Y. D. Qiu, and Y. T. Ding. 2005. Differential gene expression during capillary morphogenesis in a microcarrier-based three-dimensional in vitro model of angiogenesis with focus on chemokines and chemokine receptors. *World J Gastroenterol* 11:2283.
61. Mantovani, A., P. Allavena, and A. Sica. 2004. Tumour-associated macrophages as a prototypic type II polarised phagocyte population: role in tumour progression. *Eur J Cancer* 40:1660.
62. Mantovani, A., W. J. Ming, C. Balotta, B. Abdeljalil, and B. Bottazzi. 1986. Origin and regulation of tumor-associated macrophages: the role of tumor-derived chemotactic factor. *Biochim Biophys Acta* 865:59.
63. Leek, R. D., and A. L. Harris. 2002. Tumor-associated macrophages in breast cancer. *J Mammary Gland Biol Neoplasia* 7:177.
64. Lin, E. Y., and J. W. Pollard. 2004. Macrophages: modulators of breast cancer progression. *Novartis Found Symp* 256:158.
65. Bingle, L., C. E. Lewis, K. P. Corke, M. W. Reed, and N. J. Brown. 2006. Macrophages promote angiogenesis in human breast tumour spheroids in vivo. *Br J Cancer* 94:101.
66. Wyckoff, J., W. Wang, E. Y. Lin, Y. Wang, F. Pixley, E. R. Stanley, T. Graf, J. W. Pollard, J. Segall, and J. Condeelis. 2004. A paracrine loop between tumor cells and macrophages is required for tumor cell migration in mammary tumors. *Cancer Res* 64:7022.
67. Bolat, F., F. Kayaselcuk, T. Z. Nursal, M. C. Yagmurdur, N. Bal, and B. Demirhan. 2006. Microvessel density, VEGF expression, and tumor-associated macrophages in breast tumors: correlations with prognostic parameters. *J Exp Clin Cancer Res* 25:365.
68. Robinson, S. C., K. A. Scott, and F. R. Balkwill. 2002. Chemokine stimulation of monocyte matrix metalloproteinase-9 requires endogenous TNF-alpha. *Eur J Immunol* 32:404.
69. Klier, C. M., E. L. Nelson, C. D. Cohen, R. Horuk, D. Schlondorff, and P. J. Nelson. 2001. Chemokine-Induced secretion of gelatinase B in primary human monocytes. *Biol Chem* 382:1405.

70. Locati, M., U. Deuschle, M. L. Massardi, F. O. Martinez, M. Sironi, S. Sozzani, T. Bartfai, and A. Mantovani. 2002. Analysis of the gene expression profile activated by the CC chemokine ligand 5/RANTES and by lipopolysaccharide in human monocytes. *J Immunol* 168:3557.
71. Challita-Eid, P. M., C. N. Abboud, S. L. Morrison, M. L. Penichet, K. E. Rosell, T. Poles, S. P. Hilchey, V. Planelles, and J. D. Rosenblatt. 1998. A RANTES-antibody fusion protein retains antigen specificity and chemokine function. *J Immunol* 161:3729.
72. Manjili, M. H., H. Arnouk, K. L. Knutson, M. Kmieciak, M. L. Disis, J. R. Subjeck, and A. L. Kazim. 2006. Emergence of immune escape variant of mammary tumors that has distinct proteomic profile and a reduced ability to induce "danger signals". *Breast Cancer Res Treat* 96:233.
73. Di Carlo, E., P. Cappello, C. Sorrentino, T. D'Antuono, A. Pellicciotta, M. Giovarelli, G. Forni, P. Musiani, and F. Triebel. 2005. Immunological mechanisms elicited at the tumour site by lymphocyte activation gene-3 (LAG-3) versus IL-12: sharing a common Th1 anti-tumour immune pathway. *J Pathol* 205:82.
74. Nath, A., S. Chattopadhya, U. Chattopadhyay, and N. K. Sharma. 2006. Macrophage inflammatory protein (MIP)1alpha and MIP1beta differentially regulate release of inflammatory cytokines and generation of tumoricidal monocytes in malignancy. *Cancer Immunol Immunother* 55:1534.
75. Roda, J. M., R. Parihar, C. Magro, G. J. Nuovo, S. Tridandapani, and W. E. Carson, 3rd. 2006. Natural killer cells produce T cell-recruiting chemokines in response to antibody-coated tumor cells. *Cancer Res* 66:517.
76. Payne, A. S., and L. A. Cornelius. 2002. The role of chemokines in melanoma tumor growth and metastasis. *J Invest Dermatol* 118:915.
77. Hussein, M. R. 2005. Tumour-infiltrating lymphocytes and melanoma tumorigenesis: an insight. *Br J Dermatol* 153:18.
78. Kawakami, Y., and S. A. Rosenberg. 1997. Immunobiology of human melanoma antigens MART-1 and gp100 and their use for immuno-gene therapy. *Int Rev Immunol* 14:173.
79. Kawakami, Y., M. I. Nishimura, N. P. Restifo, S. L. Topalian, B. H. O'Neil, J. Shilyansky, J. R. Yannelli, and S. A. Rosenberg. 1993. T-cell recognition of human melanoma antigens. *J Immunother Emphasis Tumor Immunol* 14:88.
80. Lee, P. P., C. Yee, P. A. Savage, L. Fong, D. Brockstedt, J. S. Weber, D. Johnson, S. Swetter, J. Thompson, P. D. Greenberg, M. Roederer, and M. M. Davis. 1999. Characterization of circulating T cells specific for tumor-associated antigens in melanoma patients. *Nat Med* 5:677.
81. Mrowietz, U., U. Schwenk, S. Maune, J. Bartels, M. Kupper, I. Fichtner, J. M. Schroder, and D. Schadendorf. 1999. The chemokine RANTES is secreted by human melanoma cells and is associated with enhanced tumour formation in nude mice. *Br J Cancer* 79:1025.
82. Mattei, S., M. P. Colombo, C. Melani, A. Silvani, G. Parmiani, and M. Herlyn. 1994. Expression of cytokine/growth factors and their receptors in human melanoma and melanocytes. *Int J Cancer* 56:853.
83. Kershaw, M. H., G. Wang, J. A. Westwood, R. K. Pachynski, H. L. Tiffany, F. M. Marincola, E. Wang, H. A. Young, P. M. Murphy, and P. Hwu. 2002. Redirecting migration of T cells to chemokine secreted from tumors by genetic modification with CXCR2. *Hum Gene Ther* 13:1971.
84. Kunz, M., A. Toksoy, M. Goebeler, E. Engelhardt, E. Brocker, and R. Gillitzer. 1999. Strong expression of the lymphoattractant C-X-C chemokine Mig is associated with heavy infiltration of T cells in human malignant melanoma. *J Pathol* 189:552.
85. Seidl, H., E. Richtig, H. Tilz, M. Stefan, U. Schmidbauer, M. Asslaber, K. Zatloukal, M. Herlyn, and H. Schaider. 2007. Profiles of chemokine receptors in melanocytic lesions: de novo expression of CXCR6 in melanoma. *Hum Pathol* 38:768.

86. Dobrzanski, M. J., J. B. Reome, and R. W. Dutton. 2001. Immunopotentiating role of IFN-gamma in early and late stages of type 1 CD8 effector cell-mediated tumor rejection. *Clin Immunol* 98:70.
87. Mellado, M., A. M. de Ana, M. C. Moreno, C. Martinez, and J. M. Rodriguez-Frade. 2001. A potential immune escape mechanism by melanoma cells through the activation of chemokine-induced T cell death. *Curr Biol* 11:691.
88. Ng-Cashin, J., J. J. Kuhns, S. E. Burkett, J. D. Powderly, R. R. Craven, H. W. van Deventer, S. L. Kirby, and J. S. Serody. 2003. Host absence of CCR5 potentiates dendritic cell vaccination. *J Immunol* 170:4201.
89. van Deventer, H. W., W. O'Connor, Jr., W. J. Brickey, R. M. Aris, J. P. Ting, and J. S. Serody. 2005. C-C chemokine receptor 5 on stromal cells promotes pulmonary metastasis. *Cancer Res* 65:3374.
90. Wysocki, C. A., A. Panoskaltsis-Mortari, B. R. Blazar, and J. S. Serody. 2005. Leukocyte migration and graft-versus-host disease. *Blood* 105:4191.
91. Rodero, M., P. Rodero, V. Descamps, C. Lebbe, P. Wolkenstein, P. Aegerter, D. Vitoux, N. Basset-Seguin, N. Dupin, B. Grandchamp, N. Soufir, C. Combadiere, and P. Saiag. 2007. Melanoma susceptibility and progression: Association study between polymorphisms of the chemokine (CCL2) and chemokine receptors (CX3CR1, CCR5). *J Dermatol Sci* 46:72.
92. Ugurel, S., D. Schrama, G. Keller, D. Schadendorf, E. B. Brocker, R. Houben, M. Zapatka, W. Fink, H. L. Kaufman, and J. C. Becker. 2008. Impact of the CCR5 gene polymorphism on the survival of metastatic melanoma patients receiving immunotherapy. *Cancer Immunol Immunother* 57:685.
93. Padovan, E., L. Terracciano, U. Certa, B. Jacobs, A. Reschner, M. Bolli, G. C. Spagnoli, E. C. Borden, and M. Heberer. 2002. Interferon stimulated gene 15 constitutively produced by melanoma cells induces e-cadherin expression on human dendritic cells. *Cancer Res* 62:3453.
94. Chen, Z., T. Moyana, A. Saxena, R. Warrington, Z. Jia, and J. Xiang. 2001. Efficient antitumor immunity derived from maturation of dendritic cells that had phagocytosed apoptotic/necrotic tumor cells. *Int J Cancer* 93:539.
95. Kim, H. K., K. S. Song, Y. S. Park, Y. H. Kang, Y. J. Lee, K. R. Lee, K. W. Ryu, J. M. Bae, and S. Kim. 2003. Elevated levels of circulating platelet microparticles, VEGF, IL-6 and RANTES in patients with gastric cancer: possible role of a metastasis predictor. *Eur J Cancer* 39:184.
96. Fukui, R., H. Nishimori, F. Hata, T. Yasoshima, K. Ohno, H. Nomura, Y. Yanai, H. Tanaka, K. Kamiguchi, R. Denno, N. Sato, and K. Hirata. 2005. Metastases-related genes in the classification of liver and peritoneal metastasis in human gastric cancer. *J Surg Res* 129:94.
97. Hahm, K. B., Y. J. Song, T. Y. Oh, J. S. Lee, Y. J. Surh, Y. B. Kim, B. M. Yoo, J. H. Kim, S. U. Han, K. T. Nahm, M. W. Kim, D. Y. Kim, and S. W. Cho. 2003. Chemoprevention of Helicobacter pylori-associated gastric carcinogenesis in a mouse model: is it possible? *J Biochem Mol Biol* 36:82.
98. Okita, K., T. Furuhata, Y. Kimura, M. Kawakami, K. Yamaguchi, T. Tsuruma, H. Zembutsu, and K. Hirata. 2005. The interplay between gastric cancer cell lines and PBMCs mediated by the CC chemokine RANTES plays an important role in tumor progression. *J Exp Clin Cancer Res* 24:439.
99. Ohtani, N., H. Ohtani, T. Nakayama, H. Naganuma, E. Sato, T. Imai, H. Nagura, and O. Yoshie. 2004. Infiltration of CD8 + T cells containing RANTES/CCL5 + cytoplasmic granules in actively inflammatory lesions of human chronic gastritis. *Lab Invest* 84:368.
100. Burke, F., M. Relf, R. Negus, and F. Balkwill. 1996. A cytokine profile of normal and malignant ovary. *Cytokine* 8:578.
101. Melani, C., S. M. Pupa, A. Stoppacciaro, S. Menard, M. I. Colnaghi, G. Parmiani, and M. P. Colombo. 1995. An in vivo model to compare human leukocyte infiltration in carcinoma xenografts producing different chemokines. *Int J Cancer* 62:572.

102. Negus, R. P., G. W. Stamp, J. Hadley, and F. R. Balkwill. 1997. Quantitative assessment of the leukocyte infiltrate in ovarian cancer and its relationship to the expression of C-C chemokines. *Am J Pathol* 150:1723.
103. Simonitsch, I., and G. Krupitza. 1998. Autocrine self-elimination of cultured ovarian cancer cells by tumour necrosis factor alpha (TNF-alpha). *Br J Cancer* 78:862.
104. Tsukishiro, S., N. Suzumori, H. Nishikawa, A. Arakawa, and K. Suzumori. 2006. Elevated serum RANTES levels in patients with ovarian cancer correlate with the extent of the disorder. *Gynecol Oncol* 102:542.
105. Milliken, D., C. Scotton, S. Raju, F. Balkwill, and J. Wilson. 2002. Analysis of chemokines and chemokine receptor expression in ovarian cancer ascites. *Clin Cancer Res* 8:1108.
106. Dong, H. P., M. B. Elstrand, A. Holth, I. Silins, A. Berner, C. G. Trope, B. Davidson, and B. Risberg. 2006. NK- and B-cell infiltration correlates with worse outcome in metastatic ovarian carcinoma. *Am J Clin Pathol* 125:451.
107. Uekusa, Y., W. G. Yu, T. Mukai, P. Gao, N. Yamaguchi, M. Murai, K. Matsushima, S. Obika, T. Imanishi, Y. Higashibata, S. Nomura, Y. Kitamura, H. Fujiwara, and T. Hamaoka. 2002. A pivotal role for CC chemokine receptor 5 in T-cell migration to tumor sites induced by interleukin 12 treatment in tumor-bearing mice. *Cancer Res* 62:3751.
108. Hagemann, T., J. Wilson, F. Burke, H. Kulbe, N. F. Li, A. Pluddemann, K. Charles, S. Gordon, and F. R. Balkwill. 2006. Ovarian cancer cells polarize macrophages toward a tumor-associated phenotype. *J Immunol* 176:5023.
109. Yoong, K. F., S. C. Afford, R. Jones, P. Aujla, S. Qin, K. Price, S. G. Hubscher, and D. H. Adams. 1999. Expression and function of CXC and CC chemokines in human malignant liver tumors: a role for human monokine induced by gamma-interferon in lymphocyte recruitment to hepatocellular carcinoma. *Hepatology* 30:100.
110. Liu, Y., R. T. Poon, J. Hughes, X. Feng, W. C. Yu, and S. T. Fan. 2005. Chemokine receptors support infiltration of lymphocyte subpopulations in human hepatocellular carcinoma. *Clin Immunol* 114:174.
111. Liu, Y., R. T. Poon, X. Feng, W. C. Yu, J. M. Luk, and S. T. Fan. 2004. Reduced expression of chemokine receptors on peripheral blood lymphocytes in patients with hepatocellular carcinoma. *Am J Gastroenterol* 99:1111.
112. Shin, E. C., Y. H. Choi, J. S. Kim, S. J. Kim, and J. H. Park. 2002. Expression patterns of cytokines and chemokines genes in human hepatoma cells. *Yonsei Med J* 43:657.
113. Ruan, Y., Y. Guan, Z. Wu, Z. Zhang, and C. Zheng. 2003. The relationship between RANTES and mast cells recruitment in the surroundings of intrahepatic implanted tumors. *Clin Lab* 49:65.
114. Nahon, P., A. Sutton, P. Rufat, C. Faisant, C. Simon, N. Barget, J. C. Trinchet, M. Beaugrand, L. Gattegno, and N. Charnaux. 2007. Lack of association of some chemokine system polymorphisms with the risks of death and hepatocellular carcinoma occurrence in patients with alcoholic cirrhosis: a prospective study. *Eur J Gastroenterol Hepatol* 19:425.
115. Hirano, S., Y. Iwashita, A. Sasaki, S. Kai, M. Ohta, and S. Kitano. 2007. Increased mRNA expression of chemokines in hepatocellular carcinoma with tumor-infiltrating lymphocytes. *J Gastroenterol Hepatol* 22:690.
116. Lu, P., Y. Nakamoto, Y. Nemoto-Sasaki, C. Fujii, H. Wang, M. Hashii, Y. Ohmoto, S. Kaneko, K. Kobayashi, and N. Mukaida. 2003. Potential interaction between CCR1 and its ligand, CCL3, induced by endogenously produced interleukin-1 in human hepatomas. *Am J Pathol* 162:1249.

CXC Chemokines in Cancer Angiogenesis

B. Mehrad and R.M. Strieter

Abstract Chemokines were first described for their ability to recruit leukocytes, but their biological role has now been recognized in many other biological processes. Angiogenesis, or the process of new blood vessel growth, is critical to many physiologic and pathologic processes, including tumorigenesis. In this chapter, we review the role of chemokines in cancer angiogenesis and angiostasis.

Introduction

Angiogenesis, the process of growth and development of new capillaries, is a critical biological process in cancer growth. A variety of factors have been described that either promote or inhibit angiogenesis [1–14]. In the local microenvironment, net angiogenesis is determined by a balance in the expression of angiogenic, as compared to angiostatic factors. The CXC family of chemokines displays unique disparate roles in the regulation of angiogenesis. This family is structurally defined by four highly conserved cysteine amino acid residues at the NH_2-terminus, with the first two cysteines separated by a nonconserved amino acid residue [15–17]. Another structural motif further defines two subfamilies of CXC chemokines. This motif consists of a three amino acid sequence of glutamic acid-leucine-arginine (Glu-Leu-Arg; the ELR motif) immediately preceding the first cysteine amino acid residue [15–17]. Remarkably, the presence of this motif defines the angiogenic activity of CXC chemokines: CXC chemokines that contain the ELR motif promote angiogenesis [17], whereas a subset of CXC chemokines that lack the ELR motif and are inducible by interferons (IFNs) inhibits angiogenesis [17].

R.M. Strieter (✉)
Division of Pulmonary and Critical Care Medicine, Department of Medicine,
University of Virginia, Charlottesville, VA 22908, USA
e-mail: Strieter@Virginia.edu

A.M. Fulton (ed.), *Chemokine Receptors in Cancer*, Cancer Drug Discovery and Development, DOI 10.1007/978-1-60327-267-4_8,
© Humana Press, a part of Springer Science+Business Media, LLC 2009

Angiogenic CXC Chemokines

The CXC chemokine family members that promote angiogenesis are CXCL1, CXCL2, CXCL3, CXCL5, CXCL6, CXCL7, and CXCL8 (Table 1) [17]. Once released, these chemokine ligands mediate angiogenesis by several overlapping mechanisms, including promotion of endothelial cell chemotaxis, survival, and proliferation [18]. These effects are mediated via both autocrine and paracrine mechanisms; for example, vascular endothelial cell growth factor (VEGF) mediates endothelial cell expression of CXCL8 [19]. In addition, neutrophils activated by N-formyl-Met-Leu-Phe (fMLP) have been shown to release VEGF and CXCL8, thus contributing to tissue angiogenesis [20]. Furthermore, other serial pathways that promote CXC chemokine-mediated angiogenesis are operative that include receptor activation of seven-transmembrane G-protein-coupled receptors (7TM-GPCRs) and protein tyrosine kinase receptors (PTKRs) that contribute to the expression of angiogenic CXC chemokines via NF-kB activation in cancer cells and enhanced tumor-associated angiogenesis [21–24].

CXCR2: The Key Receptor for Angiogenic CXC Chemokines

In the mouse, all ELR+ CXC chemokines share a common receptor, CXCR2, whereas there are two receptors for the human ELR+ CXC chemokines, CXCR1 and CXCR2. All human ELR+ CXC chemokines can bind and signal via CXCR2, whereas only CXCL6 and CXCL8 bind specifically to CXCR1

Table 1 Human chemokine family members involved in angiogenesis

Systematic name	Human ligand	Receptor
Angiogenic		
CXCL1	Gro-α	CXCR2
CXCL2	Gro-β	CXCR2
CXCL3	Gro-γ	CXCR2
CXCL5	ENA-78	CXCR2
CXCL6	GCP-2	CXCR2
CXCL7	NAP-2	CXCR2
CXCL8	IL-8	CXCR2
CCL2	MCP-1	CCR2
Angiostatic		
CXCL4	PF-4	CXCR3B, *
CXCL4L1	PF-4 variant	CXCR3B, *
CXCL9	Mig	CXCR3B
CXCL10	IP-10	CXCR3B
CXCL11	I-TAC	CXCR3B
CXCL12	SDF-1	CXCR4
CXCL14	BRAK	?

*, additional receptors may be involved; ?, undefined receptor.

[25]. Although human endothelial cells express both CXCR1 and CXCR2 [25–27], their chemotaxis is mediated exclusively by CXCR2 and not CXCR1 [25, 26]. Exposure of human endothelial cells to CXCL8 results in phosphorylation of extracellular signal-regulated protein kinase (ERK)-1 and -2, rapid stress fiber assembly, chemotaxis, enhanced proliferation, and tube formation. Importantly, these effects can be abrogated by blocking CXCR2 with neutralizing antibodies or by inhibiting ERK-1 and ERK-2 [18].

The in vivo role of CXCR2 in mediating ELR+ CXC chemokine-induced angiogenesis has been examined in models of wound repair [28], corneal neovascularization [25], and cancer models [29]. In the wound-healing model, full-thickness excisional wounds had impaired neovascularization and slower wound healing in CXCR2-deficient mice as compared to wild-type or CXCR2+/− mice [28]. In the corneal micropocket assay of angiogenesis, both CXCR2-deficient animals and immunoneutralization of CXCR2 resulted in marked impairment of angiogenesis and corneal neovascularization [25]. Similar studies in a mouse model of implanted syngeneic nonsmall cell lung cancer (NSCLC) have shown a role for CXCR2 in mediating tumor-associated angiogenesis [29]. CXCR2-deficient hosts demonstrated reduced tumor growth and metastases, increased tumor-associated necrosis, and reduced tumor angiogenesis [29]. These in vitro and in vivo studies establish that CXCR2 is an important receptor that mediates ELR+ CXC chemokine-dependent angiogenic activity.

Ligand-bound CXCR2 is internalized and can either be targeted for degradation or be recycled to the cell surface depending on the local concentration of the ligand in relation to receptor density. Specifically, low concentrations of ligand in relation to the receptor result in sequential targeting of CXCR2 to clathrin-coated pits, early endosomes, sorting endosomes, recycling endosomes, and finally to the cell surface [30]. In contrast, prolonged or high concentrations of ELR+ CXC chemokines will result in targeting of internalized CXCR2 to late endosome and subsequently to the lysosome [30]. Importantly, CXCR2 internalization appears to be essential to chemotaxis, since inhibition of this process interrupts chemotaxis [30].

Involvement of Other Receptors in Chemokine-Mediated Angiogenesis

Given the ability of CXCR2 to mediate angiogenesis, the role of CXCR2 homologs in carcinogenesis have been investigated. Human herpes virus-8, the causative agent of Kaposi's sarcoma and primary effusive lymphoma, encodes a chemokine receptor with homology to CXCR2 [31, 32]. Similar to other chemokine receptors, this is a 7TM-GPCR and activates intracellular signaling pathways including cAMP/protein kinase A, protein kinase C, phospholipase C, phosphoinositide 3-kinase/AKT/mTOR, and NF-kB pathways [33–36]. Unlike physiologic chemokine receptors, this receptor is constitutively signaling, and its signal coupling can be further augmented by binding of ELR+ CXC chemokine ligands [37–40]. Transgenic expression of this virally encoded receptor results in development of striking focal cutaneous and visceral angioproliferative lesions that resemble the lesions of human Kaposi's sarcoma morphologically [41, 42]. In addition, transgenic expression of this viral receptor was shown to induce angiogenesis in vivo [43] and autonomous proliferation of endothelial cells in vitro [44].

The relevance of CXCR2-mediated signaling in this process was further supported by the discovery that induction of a point mutation in a highly conserved position of CXCR2 resulted in constitutive signaling and cellular transformation similar to KSHV-GPCR [31]. CXCR2 has been further identi-fied in the cellular transformation of melanocytes into melanoma [45, 46]. Therefore, the expression of CXCR2 on certain cells in the presence of persis-tent autocrine and paracrine stimulation with specific CXC chemokine ligands has important implications in promoting cellular transformation that may be relevant to the preneoplastic to neoplastic transformation in diverse neoplasms.

The red blood cell Duffy antigen (Duffy antigen receptor for chemokines, DARC) is a promiscuous but nonsignaling chemokine receptor that has the ability to act as a decoy receptor for various chemokine-mediated events [47]. In the context of angiogenesis, DARC binds the ELR+ CXC chemokine ligands CXCL1, CXCL5, and CXCL8, relevant to tumor angiogenesis [48–50]. Over-expression of this receptor in nonsmall cell tumor cell line resulted in tumor binding of ELR+ CXC chemokine ligands, thus rendering them unavailable to recruit and stimulate endothelial cells [47]. The growth of the DARC-expressing tumor cells was different from control-transfected cells in vitro. While the DARC-expressing cells formed larger tumors in vivo, these tumors displayed greater necrosis, reduced cellularity, reduced vascularity, and reduced metastatic potential in vivo [47]. These findings suggest that competitive binding of ELR+ CXC chemokines by DARC in this model can prevent paracrine activation of endothe-lial cells in the tumor microenvironment and reduce tumor-associated angiogen-esis, leading to enhanced tumor necrosis and reduced metastatic potential.

Interaction of Angiogenic CXC Chemokine Ligands with Matrix Metalloproteinases

Tumor cell invasion and metastasis is facilitated by elaboration of matrix-degrading enzymes, including serine and cysteine proteinases, and matrix metal-loproteinases. Activation of tumor cells by chemokines can result in induction of these enzymes. For example, transgenic expression of CXCL8 by a human mela-noma cell line that did not normally produce CXCL8 spontaneously resulted in upregulation of MMP-2, greater invasiveness in vitro, and increased tumor growth and metastatic potential in vivo [51]. These findings support that CXCL8 can activate tumor cell-derived collagenase activity that leads to enhanced tumor invasiveness.

CXCL8 has also been found to regulate invasiveness and metastatic potential in the context of prostate carcinoma. Overexpression of CXCL8 by prostate cancer lines results in higher metastatic potential when implanted into athymic mice, which is associated with MMP-9 expression by the cancer cells [52]. Interestingly, cells transfected with antisense CXCL8 were found to have inhibited growth and metastatic potential [52]. Similar findings were reported by another group, who found CXCL8 expression by human prostate cancer cells correlated with tumor angiogenesis and metastasis when implanted orthotopically into immunocompromised mice [53]. These findings suggest that angiogenic ELR+ CXC chemokines like CXCL8 play a multifunctional role in aiding tumor cell invasion by augmenting their local angiogenic environment and upregulating the expression of MMPs to aid tumor cell invasion and entry into the circulation.

Angiogenic CXC Chemokines in Malignancy

All angiogenic CXC chemokine genes have, in their promoter region, the ability to bind and respond to the nuclear factor-kB (NF-kB) family of transcriptional factors [17, 54, 55]. The importance of NF-kB transactivation in chemokine-mediated angiogenesis has been documented in several cancers. In the context of glioblastoma, the expression of candidate tumor-suppressor gene ING4 was recently found to be reduced in malignant cells as compared to normal brain tissue, and the extent of reduced expression correlated with tumor grade, growth rate of the tumor, and tumor-associated angiogenesis in a model system of glioblastoma implantation into immunocompromised mice [56]. The mechanism of this observation was found to relate to ING4 binding to the RelA component of NF-kB, thus inhibiting its nuclear translocation. Interestingly, this effect was entirely dependent on CXCL8, since inhibition of CXCL8 resulted in attenuated tumor growth and tumor-associated angiogenesis [56]. In further support of this concept, another study found that using a glioblastoma cell line with constitutively activated EGFR mutant leads to constitutive activation of NF-kB. Inhibition of NF-kB with a mutant IkB in these cells resulted in reduced tumor expression of CXCL8 and tumor-associated angiogenesis in vivo [57]. These data support the concept that NF-kB promotion of expression of angiogenic ELR+ CXC chemokine ligands is an important pathogenic mechanism in glioblastoma and in other cancers.

Human pancreatic cancer cell lines also secrete high levels of the angiogenic chemokines CXCL1 and CXCL8 [58, 59]. In comparing these lines using the corneal micropocket model, tumor-induced angiogenesis could be abrogated by blocking CXCR2 in tumor cells expressing high levels of angiogenic CXC chemokines [59]. The relevance of NF-kB to chemokine-mediated angiogenesis was also implicated in this context [60]; in a pancreatic cancer line with constitutive NF-kB activity, blockade of this pathway with mutant IkB resulted in reduction of tumor growth, metastatic potential, and CXCL8-mediated angiogenesis [60].

CXCL8 is also elevated in the setting of nonsmall cell lung cancer [61]. In in vivo model systems that use transplanted human nonsmall cell cancer cells in SCID mice, cell lines that constitutively express CXCL8 display greater tumorigenicity that is directly correlated to angiogenesis [62]. Tumor-derived CXCL8 correlated with tumor size and depletion of CXCL8 resulted in marked reduction in tumor growth associated with impaired angiogenesis and reduced metastatic potential [63]. Another important ELR+ CXC chemokine ligand in angiogenesis in nonsmall cell lung carcinoma is CXCL5. Correlation of CXCL5 with tumor angiogenesis was demonstrated in surgical lung cancer specimens, and levels exceeded CXCL8 [49]. In the context of in vivo animal models, immunoneutralization of CXCL5 resulted in attenuated tumor growth and spontaneous metastases, reduced angiogenesis, and augmented tumor cell apoptosis; however, CXCL5 did not influence the in vitro proliferation of the tumor cells [49]. More broadly, when all ELR+ CXC chemokines were measured in tumors in patients with nonsmall cell lung cancer, their levels correlated with patient mortality [64, 65].

Studies of CXCR2 in a lung cancer syngeneic tumor model system have shown that cancers implanted into CXCR2-deficient mice demonstrate reduced growth, increased tumor-associated necrosis, inhibited tumor-associated angiogenesis, and metastatic potential, as compared to the same tumors implanted into wild-type animals [29]. In addition, in a model of spontaneously developing lung adenocarcinomas in mice with somatic activation of the oncogene KRAS, tumors were found to produce high levels of ELR+ CXC chemokines, and neutralization of CXCR2 attenuated the development of premalignant lesions and caused apoptosis of endothelial cells, leading to reduced tumor-associated angiogenesis within the lesions [66]. In another study, the tumor expression of COX-2 was shown to mediate CXCL8 and CXCL5 production by the tumor [67]; overexpression of COX-2 by two nonsmall cancer cell lines resulted in enhanced expression of CXCL5 and CXCL8, and specific inhibition of tumor-derived COX-2 led to decreased production of these CXC chemokines. Consistent with earlier findings, in the context of a SCID mouse model of human nonsmall cell lung cancer, enhanced tumor growth of COX-2-overexpressing tumors was inhibited by neutralization of CXCL5 and CXCL8, but not VEGF [67].

The relevance of ELR+ CXC chemokines has also been studied in prostate cancer [68, 69]. Peripheral blood levels of CXCL8 are elevated in patients with prostate cancer and are highly correlated with the stage of the disease independent of prostate-specific antigen [69]. In a model of implantation of human prostate cancer into SCID mice, different prostate cancer cell lines were found to use different ELR+ CXC chemokine ligands as angiogenic mediators; in the PC-3 prostate cancer line, depletion of endogenous CXCL8 resulted in reduced tumor growth and angiogenesis, whereas in experiments with the Du145 prostate cancer line, depletion of endogenous CXCL1, but not CXCL8, resulted in a comparable effect [50]. Prostate cancer cell lines therefore appear to utilize distinct CXC chemokines to mediate their tumorigenic potential. Other studies have confirmed this observation in prostate cancer models [53].

ELR+ CXC chemokines are also important mediators in the context of malignant melanoma. CXCL1, CXCL2, and CXCL3 are highly expressed in human melanoma [45]. Transfection of genes for these ligands into immortalized murine melanocytes resulted in anchorage-independent growth in vitro and production of highly vascular tumors when implanted in immunocompromised mice [45, 46]. Neutralization of these ligands in this setting resulted in a marked reduction of tumor-derived angiogenesis and inhibition of tumor growth [45, 46], supporting the notion that these ligands act as autocrine growth factors as well as paracrine mediators of angiogenesis to promote tumorigenesis and metastases in malignant melanoma.

The progression and growth of ovarian carcinoma are also dependent on chemokine-mediated angiogenesis. In one study, the in vitro production of CXCL8 by five human ovarian cancer lines correlated with tumor neovascularization and cancer-related death when implanted into the peritoneum of immunocompromised mice, whereas VEGF production correlated only with ascites production after implantation, but basic FGF did not correlate with the outcome [70]. This concept was further substantiated in patients with ovarian cancer where ascites fluid angiogenic activity directly correlated to CXCL8 [71].

The relevance of CXCR2 ligands has also been studied in the setting of renal cell carcinoma [72]. Tumor and plasma samples from patients with metastatic renal cell carcinoma were found to have elevated levels of CXCL1, CXCL3, CXCL5, and CXCL8 as compared to healthy controls and normal tissue, respectively. In a heterotopic and orthotopic mouse models of renal cell carcinoma (RENCA), in which mouse RENCA cell line expressing GFP was injected subcutaneously into the flank or subcapsular space of the kidney, expression of CXCR2 ligands correlated with tumor volume, and the growth of the cancer was attenuated in CXCR2-deficient mice, and was associated with more necrosis of the tumor, less tumor-associated angiogenesis, and fewer metastases [72]. Similar findings have been shown in gastric carcinoma, breast, and head and neck cancer [73–77].

Angiostatic CXC Chemokines

The angiostatic ligands of the CXC chemokine family constitute a subset of the ELR-negative family members, including CXCL4, CXCL4L1, CXCL9, CXCL10, CXCL11, and CXCL14 [16, 17, 54, 78, 79] (Table 1). CXCL4 (previously designated platelet factor-4) was the first chemokine described to inhibit neovascularization [80]. A nonallelic variant of CXCL4, designated CXCL4L1, was recently isolated from activated human platelets [79]. CXCL4L1 differs from CXCL4 in only three amino acids, but is more potent for inhibiting angiogenesis in response to angiogenic stimuli [79]. CXCL4L1 has recently been shown to potently inhibit angiogenesis in the context of melanoma and nonsmall cell carcinoma in immunocompromised mice and immunocompetent mouse models [81].

CXCL9, CXCL10, and CXCL11 are unique chemokine ligands in that they are markedly induced by both type I and II IFNs [15, 82–85]. In the setting of angiogenic factors including ELR+ CXC chemokines, bFGF, and VEGF, these IFN-inducible ELR-negative CXC chemokine ligands are potent inhibitors of angiogenesis [54].

CXCL14, previously designated BRAK (breast- and kidney-expressed chemokine), is another ELR-negative CXC chemokine ligand linked to inhibition of angiogenesis [78]. CXCL14 was first identified as downregulated in head and neck squamous cell carcinoma as compared to normal oral epithelium [86]. Subsequently, CXCL14 was demonstrated to inhibit endothelial cell chemotaxis in response to CXCL8, bFGF, and VEGF, and to retard neovascularization in response to these angiogenic agonists in vivo [78]. Interestingly, CXCL14 was found to be relatively overexpressed in and around localized prostate cancers as compared to normal or hypertrophic prostate tissue, and transgenic expression of CXCL14 in a prostate cancer line and implantation into immunodeficient mice resulted in impaired cancer growth related to impaired angiogenesis [87], suggesting that in the setting of prostate cancer, CXCL14 might act as an endogenous tumor suppressor via its angiostatic properties.

CXCL12 is another ELR-negative CXC chemokine ligand implicated in tumorigenesis. While several groups have suggested that this effect might be mediated via promotion of angiogenesis via the interaction of this ligand with CXCR4 [88–91], differentiating this effect from the role of this ligand–receptor relationship in mediating metastatic spread [92] has been difficult. The argument in favor of angiogenesis is weakened by the observation that, although many tumor cells express CXCR4, CXCL12 is essentially absent from the tumor environment in breast, nonsmall cell lung, and renal cell carcinomas [92–94]. Furthermore, in the context of breast and nonsmall cell carcinomas, immunoneutralization of CXCL12 or CXCR4 did not influence tumor size or tumor-associated angiogenesis; however this intervention resulted in attenuated metastatic potential [92, 93].

CXCR3: The Main Receptor for Angiostatic CXC Chemokines

The study of specific ligand–receptor pairs in the context of angiostasis is complicated by the simultaneous expression of multiple ligands and receptors with substantial ligand–receptor redundancy. CXCR3 is the common receptor for the IFN-inducible ELR-negative CXC chemokine ligands, CXCL9, CXCL10, and CXCL11 [15, 82, 83, 95, 96]. CXCR3 exists in at least three splice variants, designated CXCR3A, CXCR3B, and CXCR3alt. CXCR3A is the major receptor found on Th1 effector T cells, cytotoxic CD8 T cells, activated B cells, and NK cells, and its expression is strongly induced by IL-2 [15, 95, 97–101]. In contrast, CXCR3B is expressed on endothelial cells and mediates the angiostatic activity of CXCL4, CXCL9, CXCL10, and CXCL11 on human microvascular endothelial cells [27, 102, 103]. The third splice variant, CXCR3alt, was described in humans and is the result of post-transcriptional exon skipping, and has a greater response to CXCL11 than CXCL9 or CXCL10 [96]. The role of CXCR3alt in angiogenesis has not been established.

Since CXCL10 contains binding domains for both CXCR3 and glycosaminoglycans, the issue of whether its angiostatic properties are mediated via binding to CXCR3 or glycosaminoglycans has recently been identified. The binding of CXCL4 and CXCL10 to cell surface heparan sulfate was originally reported to be the primary mechanism by which they inhibit endothelial cell proliferation [104]. This was addressed by generating expression constructs for mutants of CXCL10 that exhibit partial or total loss of binding to CXCR3 or with loss of binding to glycosaminoglycans but with ability to bind to CXCR3; and transfecting them into a human melanoma cell line [105]. When the resulting stable clones were introduced into immunocompromised mice, tumor lines expressing wild-type CXCL10 showed remarkable reduction in tumor growth compared to control vector-transfected tumor cells, and were essentially identical to CXCL10 mutants with partial or complete loss of glycosaminoglycans binding [105]. This work indicates that, at least in the context of this model system, tumor growth and tumor-associated angiostasis are specifically dependent on interaction of CXCL10 with CXCR3, but not glycosaminoglycans.

CXCR3-Independent Angiostatic Activity of CXCL4

The ability of CXCL4 to bind to glycosaminoglycans is important to several of its biological functions. CXCL4 inhibits endothelial cell migration, proliferation, and in vivo angiogenesis in response to bFGF or VEGF [80, 106]. Moreover, FITC-labeled CXCL4 injected systemically, selectively binds to the endothelium in only areas of active angiogenesis [107, 108]. This suggests that the microvasculature is the major target for the biological effects of CXCL4 during angiogenesis. CXCL4 has been shown to inhibit bFGF and $VEGF_{165}$ binding to their respective receptors [109–111]. One mechanism for this effect is related to the generation of CXCL4-bFGF or $CXCL4-VEGF_{165}$ heterodimeric complexes, which impairs bFGF or $VEGF_{165}$ binding to their respective receptors [110–112]. Basic FGF must undergo dimerization in the presence of endogenous heparin in order to bind to its receptor [111, 112]. CXCL4 complexes to bFGF and prevents bFGF dimerization followed by impaired receptor binding and internalization [111]. $VEGF_{165}$ possesses heparin-binding ability similar to bFGF. CXCL4 impairs $VEGF_{165}$ binding to its receptors on endothelium via a mechanism similar to what has been reported for its ability to inhibit bFGF [110].

There are additional mechanisms of CXCL4-mediated angiostatic activity, exemplified by CXCL4-mediated inhibition of angiogenesis by $VEGF_{121}$, which is not a heparin-binding protein [110, 113, 114]. In contrast to $VEGF_{165}$, CXCL4 neither forms heterodimers with $VEGF_{121}$ nor competitively interferes with

VEGF$_{121}$ binding to its receptor. These findings suggest that other mechanisms must be operative for CXCL4 inhibition of mitogen stimulation of endothelial cells, perhaps mediated through its own independent biological signal. One potential mechanism is CXCL4 inhibition of endothelial cell entry into S phase [106]. In a model system of endothelial cell stimulation independent of interaction with cell-surface glycosaminoglycans, CXCL4 inhibits epidermal growth factor (EGF)-stimulated endothelial cell proliferation by causing a decrease in cyclin E-cyclin-dependent kinase 2 (cdk2) activity that results in attenuation of retinoblastoma protein (pRb) phosphorylation [115]. The mechanism is related to CXCL4-dependent sustained increase in the levels and binding of the cyclin-dependent kinase inhibitor (CKI), p21$^{Cip1/WAF1}$, to the cyclin E-cdk2 complex. This inhibits cell cycle progression by preventing the downregulation of p21$^{Cip1/WAF1}$ leading to inhibition of both cyclin E-cdk2 activity and phosphorylation of pRb [115]. These mechanisms suggest that CXCL4 can inhibit a variety of endothelial cell mitogens at multiple levels and may be relevant to the other angiostatic ELR-negative CXC chemokines, including specific receptor binding to CXCR3.

CXCR7: A Novel CXC Chemokine Receptor

A new CXC chemokine receptor, CXCR7, has recently been identified as a novel receptor for CXCL11 and CXCL12 [116, 117]. In an early report, CXCR7 was found to be expressed by several tumor cell lines and activated endothelial cells, and its activation appears to mediate cell survival, growth, and adhesion, rather than chemotaxis [117]. Blockade of CXCR7 with a small molecule resulted in reduced tumor growth in several cancer models, including A549 human lung carcinoma xenograft in immunocompromised mice and syngeneic mouse Lewis lung carcinoma models [117]. More recently, CXCR7 was shown to be expressed on murine breast and lung carcinoma cell lines and several primary human cancers, including in tumor vasculature [118]. Overexpression of CXCR7 in a human breast cancer line resulted in formation of larger tumors in SCID mice, whereas RNAi knockdown of CXCR7 in murine breast cancer and Lewis lung carcinoma lines resulted in reduced tumor growth in syngeneic models; however the specific ligand that mediated these effects was not identified [118]. CXCR7 expression was also noted in human prostate cancer samples and corresponded with tumor aggressiveness [119]. In vitro overexpression of CXCR7 in prostate cancer cell lines resulted in increased basal proliferation and proliferation in response to CXCL12, reduced apoptotic rate, increased adherence to endothelial cell layers, and increased ability to invade matrigel, whereas reduced expression of CXCR7 by siRNA had the opposite effect [119]. Interestingly, CXCR7 overexpression also resulted in a number of downstream effects, including CXCL8 and VEGF expression by the tumor cells in vitro, and production of larger and more vascular tumors when implanted into SCID mice [119].

Interestingly, recent data suggest an antagonistic relationship between the effects of expression of CXCR4 and CXCR7 [120]. In the context of cancer, overexpressing CXCR4 by transfection in a prostate cancer cell line resulted in reduced expression of CXCR7; similarly, reducing the expression of CXCR4 by siRNA caused enhanced expression of CXCR7 [119]. In the converse, however, increased or attenuated expression of CXCR7 did not influence CXCR4 expression [119]. In summary, CXCR7 may well play an important role in mediating tumorigenesis in human cancers, but its precise contribution remains to be defined.

Angiostatic CXC Chemokines Attenuate Angiogenesis Associated with Tumorigenesis

Angiostatic CXC chemokines have been shown to inhibit angiogenesis in several tumor model systems. In the context of human nonsmall cell lung cancer, CXCL10 from resected samples was found to be significantly higher in the squamous cell carcinoma specimens than in adjacent noncancerous lung tissue or adenocarcinoma samples [121]. Interestingly, the angiostatic effects of CXCL10 were also observed in squamous cell carcinoma, in that neutralization of CXCL10 resulted in increased tumor-associated angiogenic activity. The marked difference in the levels and bioactivity of CXCL10 in squamous cell carcinoma and adenocarcinoma represents a possible mechanism for the lower patient survival, higher metastatic potential, and greater angiogenic potential observed in lung adenocarcinoma [122–124]. In a SCID mouse model, CXCL10 production from implanted adenocarcinoma and squamous cell lines correlated inversely with tumor growth, and was greater in squamous cell tumors [121]. The appearance of spontaneous lung metastases in SCID mice bearing adenocarcinoma tumors occurred after CXCL10 levels from either the primary tumor or plasma had reached a nadir [121]. In subsequent experiments, SCID mice bearing squamous cell tumors were depleted of CXCL10, whereas, animals bearing adenocarcinoma tumors were treated with intratumor CXCL10 [121]. Depletion of CXCL10 in squamous cell tumors resulted in an increase in their size [121]. In contrast, reconstitution of intratumor CXCL10 in adenocarcinoma tumors reduced both their size and metastatic potential, which was unrelated to infiltrating neutrophils or mononuclear cells (i.e., macrophages or NK cells) and directly attributable to a reduction in tumor-associated angiogenesis [121]. Similar strategies have been found for CXCL10 in melanoma using a gene therapeutic strategy [125].

In contrast to CXCL10, CXCL9 levels in human specimens of nonsmall cell carcinoma were not significantly different from that found in normal lung tissue [126]. Overexpression of CXCL9 resulted in the inhibition of NSCLC tumor growth and metastasis via a decrease in tumor-associated angiogenesis [126]. These findings support the importance of the IFN-inducible ELR-negative CXC chemokines in inhibiting nonsmall cell carcinoma growth by attenuation of tumor-derived angiogenesis. In addition, the above study demonstrated the potential efficacy of gene therapy as an alternative means to deliver and over-express a potent angiostatic CXC chemokine.

Angiostatic potential of ELR-negative chemokines has also been investi-gated in Burkitt's lymphoma cell lines in immunocompromised mice [127]. The expression of CXCL10 and CXCL9 was found to be higher in tumors that demonstrated spontaneous regression and was directly related to impaired angiogenesis [128]. To determine whether this effect was attributable to CXCL10 or CXCL9, more virulent Burkitt's lymphoma cell lines were grown in immuno-compromised mice and subjected to intratumor inoculation with either CXCL10 or CXCL9. Both conditions resulted in marked reduction in tumor-associated angiogenesis [128–131]. Although these CXCR3 ligands have been shown to bind to CXCR3 on mononuclear cells [15, 95, 97–101], the ability of these ELR-negative CXC chemokines to inhibit angiogenesis and induce lymphoma regression in immunocompromised mice supports the notion that these chemokines can med-iate their effects in a T-cell independent manner.

Immunoangiostasis: The Role of CXCR3/CXCR3 Ligand Biological Axis in Mediating Th1 Cell-Mediated Immunity and Angiostasis

Given their induction by IFNs, the expression of CXCL9, CXCL10, and CXCL11 and their angiostatic properties are closely intertwined with other immune pro-cesses, particularly of Th1 polarized immunity. Specifically, as CXCR3 ligands, CXCL9-11 represent the major chemoattractants for the recruitment of Th1 cells expressing CXCR3 during cell-mediated immunity [15, 97–100]. Thus, CXCR3 ligands play a critical role in orchestrating Th1 cytokine-induced cell-mediated immunity via the recruitment of mononuclear cells expressing CXCR3 [15, 98–100, 132].

Interestingly, Th1 cytokine-induced cell-mediated immunity and inhibition of angiogenesis appear to be interrelated in the context of nonsmall cell carci-noma [133, 134], a concept that we have described as "immunoangiostasis". Using a tumor model in immmunocompetent mice, intratumor injection of a recombinant CC chemokine, CCL21, induced complete tumor eradication in several of the treated mice [133, 134]. While CCL21-mediated antitumor responses were lymphocyte dependent, its biological effect was entirely depen-dent on the spatial generation of intratumor IFN-gamma and CXCR3 ligands [133, 134]. In immunocompetent mice, intratumoral CCL21 injection led to significant increases in CD4, CD8, NK, and dendritic cells infiltrating both the tumor and the draining lymph nodes, and a reduction in angiogenesis [133, 134]. CCL21-treated tumor-bearing mice demonstrated enhanced cytolytic capacity, suggesting the generation of a systemic immune response to tumor-associated antigens. The mononuclear cell infiltration into the tumor was associated with enhanced production of Th1 cytokines and CXCR3 ligands [133, 134]. To assess the importance of Th1 cytokines and CXCR3 ligands in mediating the effects of CCL21, depletion studies of IFN-gamma or CXCR3 ligands in the presence of CCL21 treatment demonstrated that CXCL9, CXCL10, and IFN-gamma each attenuated the antitumor effects of CCL21 [133]. These findings support the notion that CCL21-mediated antitumor response was CXCR3 ligand dependent. These findings are similar to the previously reported study of IL-12-mediated regression of RENCA in a murine model, where the anti-tumor effect of IL-12 was lost when CXCR3 ligands were depleted [135]. More recently, the effectiveness of systemic IL-2 therapy in the mouse model of RENCA was shown to be CXCR3 dependent, and resulted in upregulation of CXCR3 on peripheral blood mononuclear cells, but, surprisingly, downregulation of CXCR3 ligands in the tumor [136]. The effectiveness of this therapy was substantially enhanced when it was combined with overexpression of the CXCR3 ligand, CXCL9, in the tumor [136]. The mechanism for inhibition of tumor growth was related to both attenuation of tumor-associated angiogenesis and enhanced immunity toward specific tumor-associated antigens [136]. These findings support the notion that CXCR3 and its ligands contribute to antitumor defenses by two distinct and additive mechanisms, namely inhibition of angiogenesis and mediating direct antitumor immunity.

Conclusion

Although CXC chemokine biology was originally felt to be restricted to recruitment of subpopulations of leukocytes, it has become increasingly clear that these cytokines can display pleiotropic effects in mediating biology that goes beyond their originally described function. CXC chemokines are a unique cytokine family that exhibit on the basis of structure/function and receptor binding/activation either angiogenic or angiostatic biological activity in the regulation of angiogenesis. CXC chemokines appear to be important in the regulation of angiogenesis associated with both tumorigenesis and the pathogenesis of chronic inflammatory/fibroproliferative disorders. These findings support the notion that therapy directed at either inhibition of angiogenic or augmentation of angiostatic CXC chemokines may be a novel approach in the treatment of a variety of disorders associated with aberrant angiogenesis.

Acknowledgments This work was supported by NIH grants HL73848 and an American Lung Association Career Investigator Award (Mehrad) and CA87879 and HL66027 (Strieter).

References

1. Auerbach, W. and R. Auerbach. Angiogenesis inhibition: a review. Pharmacol Ther *63*: 265–311, 1994.
2. Auerbach, R., W. Auerbach, and I. Polakowski. Assays for angiogenesis: a review. Pharmacol Ther *51*: 1–11, 1991.

3. Ziche, M., L. Morbidelli, and S. Donnini. Angiogenesis. Exp Nephrol *4*: 1–14, 1996.
4. Pluda, J.M. Tumor-associated angiogenesis: mechanisms, clinical implications, and therapeutic strategies. Semin Oncol *24*: 203–18, 1997.
5. Pluda, J.M. and D.R. Parkinson. Clinical implications of tumor-associated neovascularization and current antiangiogenic strategies for the treatment of malignancies of pancreas. Cancer *78*: 680–7, 1996.
6. Gastl, G., T. Hermann, M. Steurer, J. Zmija, E. Gunsilius, C. Unger, and A. Kraft. Angiogenesis as a target for tumor treatment. Oncology *54*: 177–84, 1997.
7. Risau, W. Angiogenesis is coming of age. Circ Res *82*: 926–8, 1998.
8. Risau, W. Mechanisms of angiogenesis. Nature *386*: 671–4, 1997.
9. Hotfilder, M., U. Nowak-Gottl, and J.E. Wolff. Tumorangiogenesis: a network of cytokines. Klin Padiatr *209*: 265–70, 1997.
10. Hui, Y.F. and R.J. Ignoffo. Angiogenesis inhibitors. A promising role in cancer therapy. Cancer Pract *6*: 60–2, 1998.
11. Kumar, R. and I.J. Fidler. Angiogenic molecules and cancer metastasis. In Vivo *12*: 27–34, 1998.
12. Zetter, B.R. Angiogenesis. State of the art. Chest *93*: 159S–166S, 1988.
13. Zetter, B.R. Angiogenesis and tumor metastasis. Annu Rev Med *49*: 407–24, 1998.
14. Lund, E.L., M. Spang-Thomsen, H. Skovgaard-Poulsen, and P.E. Kristjansen. Tumor angiogenesis–a new therapeutic target in gliomas. Acta Neurol Scand *97*: 52–62, 1998.
15. Luster, A.D. Chemokines–chemotactic cytokines that mediate inflammation. N Engl J Med *338*: 436–45, 1998.
16. Belperio, J.A., M.P. Keane, D.A. Arenberg, C.L. Addison, J.E. Ehlert, M.D. Burdick, and R.M. Strieter. CXC chemokines in angiogenesis. J Leukoc Biol *68*: 1–8, 2000.
17. Strieter, R.M., P.J. Polverini, S.L. Kunkel, D.A. Arenberg, M.D. Burdick, J. Kasper, J. Dzuiba, J.V. Damme, A. Walz, D. Marriott, S.Y. Chan, S. Roczniak, and A.B. Shanafelt. The functional role of the 'ELR' motif in CXC chemokine-mediated angiogenesis. J Biol Chem *270*: 27348–57, 1995.
18. Heidemann, J., H. Ogawa, M.B. Dwinell, P. Rafiee, C. Maaser, H.R. Gockel, M.F. Otterson, D.M. Ota, N. Lugering, W. Domschke, and D.G. Binion. Angiogenic effects of interleukin 8 (CXCL8) in human intestinal microvascular endothelial cells are mediated by CXCR2. J Biol Chem *278*: 8508–15, 2003.
19. Nor, J.E., J. Christensen, J. Liu, M. Peters, D.J. Mooney, R.M. Strieter, and P.J. Polverini. Up-Regulation of Bcl-2 in microvascular endothelial cells enhances intratumoral angiogenesis and accelerates tumor growth. Cancer Res *61*: 2183–8., 2001.
20. Schruefer, R., N. Lutze, J. Schymeinsky, and B. Walzog. Human neutrophils promote angiogenesis by a paracrine feedforward mechanism involving endothelial interleukin-8. Am J Physiol Heart Circ Physiol *288*: H1186–92, 2005.
21. Dong, G., Z. Chen, Z.Y. Li, N.T. Yeh, C.C. Bancroft, and C. Van Waes. Hepatocyte growth factor/scatter factor-induced activation of MEK and PI3K signal pathways contributes to expression of proangiogenic cytokines interleukin-8 and vascular endothelial growth factor in head and neck squamous cell carcinoma. Cancer Res *61*: 5911–8, 2001.
22. Hirata, A., S. Ogawa, T. Kometani, T. Kuwano, S. Naito, M. Kuwano, and M. Ono. ZD1839 (Iressa) induces antiangiogenic effects through inhibition of epidermal growth factor receptor tyrosine kinase. Cancer Res *62*: 2554–60, 2002.
23. Levine, L., J.A. Lucci, 3rd, B. Pazdrak, J.Z. Cheng, Y.S. Guo, C.M. Townsend, Jr., and M.R. Hellmich. Bombesin stimulates nuclear factor kappa B activation and expression of proangiogenic factors in prostate cancer cells. Cancer Res *63*: 3495–502, 2003.
24. Richmond, A. Nf-kappa B, chemokine gene transcription and tumour growth. Nat Rev Immunol *2*: 664–74, 2002.
25. Addison, C.L., T.O. Daniel, M.D. Burdick, H. Liu, J.E. Ehlert, Y.Y. Xue, L. Buechi, A. Walz, A. Richmond, and R.M. Strieter. The CXC chemokine receptor 2, CXCR2, is the

putative receptor for ELR(+) CXC chemokine-induced angiogenic activity J Immunol *165*: 5269–77, 2000.

26. Murdoch, C., P.N. Monk, and A. Finn. CXC Chemokine receptor expression on human endothelial cells. Cytokine *11*: 704–712, 1999.

27. Salcedo, R., J.H. Resau, D. Halverson, E.A. Hudson, M. Dambach, D. Powell, K. Wasserman, and J.J. Oppenheim. Differential expression and responsiveness of chemokine receptors (CXCR1–3) by human microvascular endothelial cells and umbilical vein endothelial cells. Faseb J *14*: 2055–64, 2000.

28. Devalaraja, R.M., L.B. Nanney, J. Du, Q. Qian, Y. Yu, M.N. Devalaraja, and A. Richmond. Delayed wound healing in CXCR2 knockout mice. J Invest Dermatol *115*: 234–44, 2000.

29. Keane, M.P., J.A. Belperio, Y.Y. Xue, M.D. Burdick, and R.M. Strieter. Depletion of CXCR2 inhibits tumor growth and angiogenesis in a murine model of lung cancer. J Immunol *172*: 2853–60, 2004.

30. Richmond, A., G.H. Fan, P. Dhawan, and J. Yang. How do chemokine/chemokine receptor activations affect tumorigenesis? Novartis Found Symp *256*: 74–89; discussion 89–91, 106–11, 266–9, 2004.

31. Burger, M., J.A. Burger, R.C. Hoch, Z. Oades, H. Takamori, and I.U. Schraufstatter. Point mutation causing constitutive signaling of CXCR2 leads to transforming activity similar to Kaposi's sarcoma herpesvirus-G protein- coupled receptor. J Immunol *163*: 2017–22, 1999.

32. Gershengorn, M.C., E. Geras-Raaka, A. Varma, and I. Clark-Lewis. Chemokines activate Kaposi's sarcoma-associated herpesvirus G protein- coupled receptor in mammalian cells in culture. J Clin Invest *102*: 1469–72, 1998.

33. Sugden, P.H. and A. Clerk. Regulation of the ERK subgroup of MAP kinase cascades through G protein- coupled receptors. Cell Signal *9*: 337–51, 1997.

34. Pawson, T. and J.D. Scott. Signaling through scaffold, anchoring, and adaptor proteins. Science *278*: 2075–80, 1997.

35. Shyamala, V. and H. Khoja. Interleukin-8 receptors R1 and R2 activate mitogen-activated protein kinases and induce c-fos, independent of Ras and Raf-1 in Chinese hamster ovary cells. Biochemistry *37*: 15918–24, 1998.

36. Couty, J.P. and M.C. Gershengorn. Insights into the viral G protein-coupled receptor encoded by human herpesvirus type 8 (HHV-8). Biol Cell *96*: 349–54, 2004.

37. Arvanitakis, L., E. Geras-Raaka, A. Varma, M.C. Gershengorn, and E. Cesarman. Human herpesvirus KSHV encodes a constitutively active G-protein- coupled receptor linked to cell proliferation. Nature *385*: 347–50, 1997.

38. Bais, C., B. Santomasso, O. Coso, L. Arvanitakis, E.G. Raaka, J.S. Gutkind, A.S. Asch, E. Cesarman, M.C. Gershengorn, E.A. Mesri, and M.C. Gerhengorn. G-protein-coupled receptor of Kaposi's sarcoma-associated herpesvirus is a viral oncogene and angiogenesis activator. Nature *391*: 86–9, 1998.

39. Geras-Raaka, E., L. Arvanitakis, C. Bais, E. Cesarman, E.A. Mesri, and M.C. Gershengorn. Inhibition of constitutive signaling of Kaposi's sarcoma-associated herpesvirus G protein-coupled receptor by protein kinases in mammalian cells in culture. J Exp Med *187*: 801–6, 1998.

40. Geras-Raaka, E., A. Varma, H. Ho, I. Clark-Lewis, and M.C. Gershengorn. Human interferon-gamma-inducible protein 10 (IP-10) inhibits constitutive signaling of Kaposi's sarcoma-associated herpesvirus G protein-coupled receptor. J Exp Med *188*: 405–8, 1998.

41. Yang, T.Y., S.C. Chen, M.W. Leach, D. Manfra, B. Homey, M. Wiekowski, L. Sullivan, C.H. Jenh, S.K. Narula, S.W. Chensue, and S.A. Lira. Transgenic expression of the chemokine receptor encoded by human herpesvirus 8 induces an angioproliferative disease resembling Kaposi's sarcoma. J Exp Med *191*: 445–54, 2000.

42. Guo, H.G., M. Sadowska, W. Reid, E. Tschachler, G. Hayward, and M. Reitz. Kaposi's sarcoma-like tumors in a human herpesvirus 8 ORF74 transgenic mouse. J Virol 77: 2631–9, 2003.
43. Jensen, K.K., D.J. Manfra, M.G. Grisotto, A.P. Martin, G. Vassileva, K. Kelley, T.W. Schwartz, and S.A. Lira. The human herpes virus 8-encoded chemokine receptor is required for angioproliferation in a murine model of Kaposi's sarcoma. J Immunol 174: 3686–94, 2005.
44. Grisotto, M.G., A. Garin, A.P. Martin, K.K. Jensen, P. Chan, S.C. Sealfon, and S.A. Lira. The human herpesvirus 8 chemokine receptor vGPCR triggers autonomous proliferation of endothelial cells. J Clin Invest 116: 1264–73, 2006.
45. Luan, J., R. Shattuck-Brandt, H. Haghnegahdar, J.D. Owen, R. Strieter, M. Burdick, C. Nirodi, D. Beauchamp, K.N. Johnson, and A. Richmond. Mechanism and biological significance of constitutive expression of MGSA/GRO chemokines in malignant melanoma tumor progression. J Leukoc Biol 62: 588–97, 1997.
46. Owen, J.D., R. Strieter, M. Burdick, H. Haghnegahdar, L. Nanney, R. Shattuck-Brandt, and A. Richmond. Enhanced tumor-forming capacity for immortalized melanocytes expressing melanoma growth stimulatory activity/growth-regulated cytokine beta and gamma proteins. Int J Cancer 73: 94–103, 1997.
47. Addison, C.L., J.A. Belperio, M.D. Burdick, and R.M. Strieter. Overexpression of the duffy antigen receptor for chemokines (DARC) by NSCLC tumor cells results in increased tumor necrosis. BMC Cancer 4: 28, 2004.
48. Arenberg, D.A., S.L. Kunkel, P.J. Polverini, M. Glass, M.D. Burdick, and R.M. Strieter. Inhibition of interleukin-8 reduces tumorigenesis of human non-small cell lung cancer in SCID mice. J Clin Invest 97: 2792–802, 1996.
49. Arenberg, D.A., M.P. Keane, B. DiGiovine, S.L. Kunkel, S.B. Morris, Y.Y. Xue, M.D. Burdick, M.C. Glass, M.D. Iannettoni, and R.M. Strieter. Epithelial-neutrophil activating peptide (ENA-78) is an important angiogenic factor in non-small cell lung cancer. J Clin Invest 102: 465–72, 1998.
50. Moore, B.B., D.A. Arenberg, K. Stoy, T. Morgan, C.L. Addison, S.B. Morris, M. Glass, C. Wilke, Y.Y. Xue, S. Sitterding, S.L. Kunkel, M.D. Burdick, and R.M. Strieter. Distinct CXC chemokines mediate tumorigenicity of prostate cancer cells. Am J Pathol 154: 1503–12, 1999.
51. Luca, M., S. Huang, J.E. Gershenwald, R.K. Singh, R. Reich, and M. Bar-Eli. Expression of interleukin-8 by human melanoma cells up-regulates MMP-2 activity and increases tumor growth and metastasis. Am J Pathol 151: 1105–13, 1997.
52. Inoue, K., J.W. Slaton, B.Y. Eve, S.J. Kim, P. Perrotte, M.D. Balbay, S. Yano, M. Bar-Eli, R. Radinsky, C.A. Pettaway, and C.P. Dinney. Interleukin 8 expression regulates tumorigenicity and metastases in androgen-independent prostate cancer. Clin Cancer Res 6: 2104–19, 2000.
53. Kim, S.J., H. Uehara, T. Karashima, M. McCarty, N. Shih, and I.J. Fidler. Expression of interleukin-8 correlates with angiogenesis, tumorigenicity, and metastasis of human prostate cancer cells implanted orthotopically in nude mice. Neoplasia 3: 33–42, 2001.
54. Strieter, R.M., J.A. Belperio, D.A. Arenberg, M.I. Smith, M.D. Burdick, and M.P. Keane. "CXC chemokine in angiogenesis," in Chemokines and the Nervous System, ed. Ransohoff, R.M., K. Suzuki, A.E.I. Proudfoot and W.F. Hickey (Amsterdam, The Netherlands: Elsevier Science B.V., 2002).
55. Ghosh, S., M.J. May, and E.B. Kopp. NF-kappa B and Rel proteins: evolutionarily conserved mediators of immune responses. Annu Rev Immunol 16: 225–60, 1998.
56. Garkavtsev, I., S.V. Kozin, O. Chernova, L. Xu, F. Winkler, E. Brown, G.H. Barnett, and R.K. Jain. The candidate tumour suppressor protein ING4 regulates brain tumour growth and angiogenesis. Nature 428: 328–32, 2004.

57. Wu, J.L., T. Abe, R. Inoue, M. Fujiki, and H. Kobayashi. IkappaBalphaM suppresses angiogenesis and tumorigenesis promoted by a constitutively active mutant EGFR in human glioma cells. Neurol Res 26: 785–91, 2004.

58. Takamori, H., Z.G. Oades, O.C. Hoch, M. Burger, and I.U. Schraufstatter. Autocrine growth effect of IL-8 and GROalpha on a human pancreatic cancer cell line, Capan-1. Pancreas 21: 52–6, 2000.

59. Wente, M.N., M.P. Keane, M.D. Burdick, H. Friess, M.W. Buchler, G.O. Ceyhan, H.A. Reber, R.M. Strieter, and O.J. Hines. Blockade of the chemokine receptor CXCR2 inhibits pancreatic cancer cell-induced angiogenesis. Cancer Lett 241: 221–7, 2006.

60. Xiong, H.Q., J.L. Abbruzzese, E. Lin, L. Wang, L. Zheng, and K. Xie. NF-kappaB activity blockade impairs the angiogenic potential of human pancreatic cancer cells. Int J Cancer 108: 181–8, 2004.

61. Smith, D.R., P.J. Polverini, S.L. Kunkel, M.B. Orringer, R.I. Whyte, M.D. Burdick, C.A. Wilke, and R.M. Strieter. IL-8 mediated angiogenesis in human bronchogenic carcinoma. J. Exp. Med. 179: 1409–1415, 1994.

62. Yatsunami, J., N. Tsuruta, K. Ogata, K. Wakamatsu, K. Takayama, M. Kawasaki, Y. Nakanishi, N. Hara, and S. Hayashi. Interleukin-8 participates in angiogenesis in non-small cell, but not small cell carcinoma of the lung. Cancer Lett 120: 101–8, 1997.

63. Arenberg, D.A., S.L. Kunkel, M.D. Burdick, P.J. Polverini, and R.M. Strieter. Treatment with anti-IL-8 inhibits non-small cell lung cancer tumor growth (Meeting abstract). J Invest Med 43: 479A 1995, 1995.

64. White, E.S., K.R. Flaherty, S. Carskadon, A. Brant, M.D. Iannettoni, J. Yee, M.B. Orringer, and D.A. Arenberg. Macrophage migration inhibitory factor and CXC chemokine expression in non-small cell lung cancer: role in angiogenesis and prognosis. Clin Cancer Res 9: 853–60, 2003.

65. Chen, J.J., P.L. Yao, A. Yuan, T.M. Hong, C.T. Shun, M.L. Kuo, Y.C. Lee, and P.C. Yang. Up-regulation of tumor interleukin-8 expression by infiltrating macrophages: its correlation with tumor angiogenesis and patient survival in non-small cell lung cancer. Clin Cancer Res 9: 729–37, 2003.

66. Wislez, M., N. Fujimoto, J.G. Izzo, A.E. Hanna, D.D. Cody, R.R. Langley, H. Tang, M.D. Burdick, M. Sato, J.D. Minna, L. Mao, I. Wistuba, R.M. Strieter, and J.M. Kurie. High expression of ligands for chemokine receptor CXCR2 in alveolar epithelial neoplasia induced by oncogenic kras. Cancer Res 66: 4198–207, 2006.

67. Pold, M., L.X. Zhu, S. Sharma, M.D. Burdick, Y. Lin, P.P. Lee, A. Pold, J. Luo, K. Krysan, M. Dohadwala, J.T. Mao, R.K. Batra, R.M. Strieter, and S.M. Dubinett. Cyclooxygenase-2-dependent expression of angiogenic CXC chemokines ENA-78/CXC Ligand (CXCL) 5 and interleukin-8/CXCL8 in human non-small cell lung cancer. Cancer Res 64: 1853–60, 2004.

68. Bostwick, D.G. and K.A. Iczkowski. Microvessel density in prostate cancer: prognostic and therapeutic utility. Semin Urol Oncol 16: 118–23, 1998.

69. Fregene, T.A., P.S. Khanuja, A.C. Noto, S.K. Gehani, E.M. Van Egmont, D.A. Luz, and K.J. Pienta. Tumor-associated angiogenesis in prostate cancer. Anticancer Res 13: 2377–81, 1993.

70. Yoneda, J., H. Kuniyasu, M.A. Crispens, J.E. Price, C.D. Bucana, and I.J. Fidler. Expression of angiogenesis-related genes and progression of human ovarian carcinomas in nude mice. J Natl Cancer Inst 90: 447–54, 1998.

71. Gawrychowski, K., E. Skopinska-Rozewska, E. Barcz, E. Sommer, B. Szaniawska, K. Roszkowska-Purska, P. Janik, and J. Zielinski Angiogenic activity and interleukin-8 content of human ovarian cancer ascites. Eur J Gynaecol Oncol 19: 262–4, 1998.

72. Mestas, J., M.D. Burdick, K. Reckamp, A. Pantuck, R.A. Figlin, and R.M. Strieter. The role of CXCR2/CXCR2 ligand biological axis in renal cell carcinoma. J Immunol 175: 5351–7, 2005.

73. Miller, L.J., S.H. Kurtzman, Y. Wang, K.H. Anderson, R.R. Lindquist, and D.L. Kreutzer. Expression of interleukin-8 receptors on tumor cells and vascular endothelial cells in human breast cancer tissue. Anticancer Res *18*: 77–81, 1998.
74. Richards, B.L., R.J. Eisma, J.D. Spiro, R.L. Lindquist, and D.L. Kreutzer. Coexpression of interleukin-8 receptors in head and neck squamous cell carcinoma. Am J Surg *174*: 507–12, 1997.
75. Singh, R.K., M. Gutman, R. Radinsky, C.D. Bucana, and I.J. Fidler. Expression of interleukin 8 correlates with the metastatic potential of human melanoma cells in nude mice. Cancer Res *54*: 3242–7, 1994.
76. Cohen, R.F., J. Contrino, J.D. Spiro, E.A. Mann, L.L. Chen, and D.L. Kreutzer. Interleukin-8 expression by head and neck squamous cell carcinoma. Arch Otolaryngol Head Neck Surg *121*: 202–9, 1995.
77. Chen, Z., P.S. Malhotra, G.R. Thomas, F.G. Ondrey, D.C. Duffey, C.W. Smith, I. Enamorado, N.T. Yeh, G.S. Kroog, S. Rudy, L. McCullagh, S. Mousa, M. Quezado, L.L. Herscher, and C. Van Waes. Expression of proinflammatory and proangiogenic cytokines in patients with head and neck cancer. Clin Cancer Res *5*: 1369–79, 1999.
78. Shellenberger, T.D., M. Wang, M. Gujrati, A. Jayakumar, R.M. Strieter, C. Ioannides, C.L. Efferson, A.K. El-Naggar, G.L. Clayman, and M.J. Frederick. BRAK/CXCL14 is a potent inhibitor of angiogenesis and is a chemotactic factor for immature dendritic cells. Cancer Res. *64*: 8262–8270, 2004.
79. Struyf, S., M.D. Burdick, P. Proost, J. Van Damme, and R.M. Strieter. Platelets release CXCL4L1, a nonallelic variant of the chemokine platelet factor-4/CXCL4 and potent inhibitor of angiogenesis. Circ Res *95*: 855–7, 2004.
80. Maione, T.E., G.S. Gray, J. Petro, A.J. Hunt, A.L. Donner, S.I. Bauer, H.F. Carson, and R.J. Sharpe. Inhibition of angiogenesis by recombinant human platelet factor-4 and related peptides. Science *247*: 77–9, 1990.
81. Struyf, S., M.D. Burdick, E. Peeters, K. Van den Broeck, C. Dillen, P. Proost, J. Van Damme, and R.M. Strieter. Platelet factor-4 variant chemokine CXCL4L1 inhibits melanoma and lung carcinoma growth and metastasis by preventing angiogenesis. Cancer Res *67*: 5940–8, 2007.
82. Rollins, B.J. Chemokines. Blood *90*: 909–28, 1997.
83. Balkwill, F. The molecular and cellular biology of the chemokines. J Viral Hepat *5*: 1–14, 1998.
84. Strieter, R.M., J.A. Belperio, R.J. Phillips, and M.P. Keane. Chemokines: angiogenesis and metastases in lung cancer. Novartis Found Symp *256*: 173–84; discussion 184–8, 259–69, 2004.
85. Strieter, R.M., J.A. Belperio, R.J. Phillips, and M.P. Keane. CXC chemokines in angiogenesis of cancer. Semin Cancer Biol *14*: 195–200, 2004.
86. Frederick, M.J., Y. Henderson, X. Xu, M.T. Deavers, A.A. Sahin, H. Wu, D.E. Lewis, A.K. El-Naggar, and G.L. Clayman. In vivo expression of the novel CXC chemokine BRAK in normal and cancerous human tissue. Am J Pathol *156*: 1937–50, 2000.
87. Schwarze, S.R., J. Luo, W.B. Isaacs, and D.F. Jarrard. Modulation of CXCL14 (BRAK) expression in prostate cancer. Prostate *13*: 13, 2005.
88. Bachelder, R.E., M.A. Wendt, and A.M. Mercurio. Vascular endothelial growth factor promotes breast carcinoma invasion in an autocrine manner by regulating the chemokine receptor CXCR4. Cancer Res *62*: 7203–6, 2002.
89. Salcedo, R. and J.J. Oppenheim. Role of chemokines in angiogenesis: CXCL12/SDF-1 and CXCR4 interaction, a key regulator of endothelial cell responses. Microcirculation *10*: 359–70, 2003.
90. Kijowski, J., M. Baj-Krzyworzeka, M. Majka, R. Reca, L.A. Marquez, M. Christofidou-Solomidou, A. Janowska-Wieczorek, and M.Z. Ratajczak. The SDF-1-CXCR4 axis stimulates VEGF secretion and activates integrins but does not affect proliferation and survival in lymphohematopoietic cells. Stem Cells *19*: 453–66, 2001.

91. Salcedo, R., K. Wasserman, H.A. Young, M.C. Grimm, O.M. Howard, M.R. Anver, H.K. Kleinman, W.J. Murphy, and J.J. Oppenheim. Vascular endothelial growth factor and basic fibroblast growth factor induce expression of CXCR4 on human endothelial cells: In vivo neovascularization induced by stromal-derived factor-1alpha. Am J Pathol *154*: 1125–35, 1999.

92. Phillips, R.J., M.D. Burdick, M. Lutz, J.A. Belperio, M.P. Keane, and R.M. Strieter. The stromal derived factor-1/CXCL12-CXC chemokine receptor 4 biological axis in non-small cell lung cancer metastases. Am J Respir Crit Care Med *167*: 1676–86, 2003.

93. Muller, A., B. Homey, H. Soto, N. Ge, D. Catron, M.E. Buchanan, T. McClanahan, E. Murphy, W. Yuan, S.N. Wagner, J.L. Barrera, A. Mohar, E. Verastegui, and A. Zlotnik. Involvement of chemokine receptors in breast cancer metastasis. Nature *410*: 50–6, 2001.

94. Schrader, A.J., O. Lechner, M. Templin, K.E. Dittmar, S. Machtens, M. Mengel, M. Probst-Kepper, A. Franzke, T. Wollensak, P. Gatzlaff, J. Atzpodien, J. Buer, and J. Lauber. CXCR4/CXCL12 expression and signalling in kidney cancer. Br J Cancer *86*: 1250–6, 2002.

95. Loetscher, M., P. Loetscher, N. Brass, E. Meese, and B. Moser. Lymphocyte-specific chemokine receptor CXCR3: regulation, chemokine binding and gene localization. Eur J Immunol *28*: 3696–705, 1998.

96. Ehlert, J.E., C.A. Addison, M.D. Burdick, S.L. Kunkel, and R.M. Strieter. identification and partial characterization of a variant of human CXCR3 generated by posttranscriptional exon skipping. J Immunol *173*: 6234–6240, 2004.

97. Moser, B. and P. Loetscher. Lymphocyte traffic control by chemokines. Nat Immunol *2*: 123–8, 2001.

98. Loetscher, M., B. Gerber, P. Loetscher, S.A. Jones, L. Piali, I. Clark-Lewis, M. Baggiolini, and B. Moser. Chemokine receptor specific for IP10 and mig: structure, function, and expression in activated T-lymphocytes. J Exp Med *184*: 963–9, 1996.

99. Rabin, R.L., M.K. Park, F. Liao, R. Swofford, D. Stephany, and J.M. Farber. Chemokine receptor responses on T cells are achieved through regulation of both receptor expression and signaling. J Immunol *162*: 3840–50, 1999.

100. Qin, S., J.B. Rottman, P. Myers, N. Kassam, M. Weinblatt, M. Loetscher, A.E. Koch, B. Moser, and C.R. Mackay. The chemokine receptors CXCR3 and CCR5 mark subsets of T cells associated with certain inflammatory reactions. J Clin Invest *101*: 746–54, 1998.

101. Beider, K., A. Nagler, O. Wald, S. Franitza, M. Dagan-Berger, H. Wald, H. Giladi, S. Brocke, J. Hanna, O. Mandelboim, M. Darash-Yahana, E. Galun, and A. Peled. Involvement of CXCR4 and IL-2 in the homing and retention of human NK and NK T cells to the bone marrow and spleen of NOD/SCID mice. Blood *102*: 1951–8, 2003.

102. Romagnani, P., F. Annunziato, L. Lasagni, E. Lazzeri, C. Beltrame, M. Francalanci, M. Uguccioni, G. Galli, L. Cosmi, L. Maurenzig, M. Baggiolini, E. Maggi, S. Romagnani, and M. Serio. Cell cycle-dependent expression of CXC chemokine receptor 3 by endothelial cells mediates angiostatic activity. J Clin Invest *107*: 53–63, 2001.

103. Lasagni, L., M. Francalanci, F. Annunziato, E. Lazzeri, S. Giannini, L. Cosmi, C. Sagrinati, B. Mazzinghi, C. Orlando, E. Maggi, F. Marra, S. Romagnani, M. Serio, and P. Romagnani. An alternatively spliced variant of CXCR3 mediates the inhibition of endothelial cell growth induced by IP-10, Mig, and I-TAC, and acts as functional receptor for platelet factor 4. J Exp Med *197*: 1537–49, 2003.

104. Luster, A.D., S.M. Greenberg, and P. Leder. The IP-10 chemokine binds to a specific cell surface heparan sulfate site shared with platelet factor 4 and inhibits endothelial cell proliferation. J Exp Med *182*: 219–31, 1995.

105. Yang, J. and A. Richmond. The angiostatic activity of interferon-inducible protein-10/CXCL10 in human melanoma depends on binding to CXCR3 but not to glycosaminoglycan. Mol Ther *9*: 846–55, 2004.

106. Gupta, S.K. and J.P. Singh. Inhibition of endothelial cell proliferation by platelet factor-4 involves a unique action on S phase progression. J Cell Biol *127*: 1121–7, 1994.

107. Hansell, P., T.E. Maione, and P. Borgstrom. Selective binding of platelet factor 4 to regions of active angiogenesis in vivo. Am J Physiol *269*: H829–36, 1995.

108. Borgstrom, P., R. Discipio, and T.E. Maione. Recombinant platelet factor 4, an angiogenic marker for human breast carcinoma. Anticancer Res *18*: 4035–41, 1998.

109. Sato, Y., M. Abe, and R. Takaki. Platelet factor 4 blocks the binding of basic fibroblast growth factor to the receptor and inhibits the spontaneous migration of vascular endothelial cells. Biochem Biophys Res Commun *172*: 595–600, 1990.

110. Gengrinovitch, S., S.M. Greenberg, T. Cohen, H. Gitay-Goren, P. Rockwell, T.E. Maione, B.Z. Levi, and G. Neufeld. Platelet factor-4 inhibits the mitogenic activity of VEGF121 and VEGF165 using several concurrent mechanisms. J Biol Chem *270*: 15059–65, 1995.

111. Perollet, C., Z.C. Han, C. Savona, J.P. Caen, and A. Bikfalvi. Platelet factor 4 modulates fibroblast growth factor 2 (FGF-2) activity and inhibits FGF-2 dimerization. Blood *91*: 3289–99, 1998.

112. Jouan, V., X. Canron, M. Alemany, J.P. Caen, G. Quentin, J. Plouet, and A. Bikfalvi Inhibition of in vitro angiogenesis by platelet factor-4-derived peptides and mechanism of action. Blood *94*: 984–93, 1999.

113. Houck, K.A., D.W. Leung, A.M. Rowland, J. Winer, and N. Ferrara. Dual regulation of vascular endothelial growth factor bioavailability by genetic and proteolytic mechanisms. J Biol Chem *267*: 26031–7, 1992.

114. Houck, K.A., N. Ferrara, J. Winer, G. Cachianes, B. Li, and D.W. Leung. The vascular endothelial growth factor family: identification of a fourth molecular species and characterization of alternative splicing of RNA. Mol Endocrinol *5*: 1806–14, 1991.

115. Gentilini, G., N.E. Kirschbaum, J.A. Augustine, R.H. Aster, and G.P. Visentin. Inhibition of human umbilical vein endothelial cell proliferation by the CXC chemokine, platelet factor 4 (PF4), is associated with impaired downregulation of p21(Cip1/WAF1). Blood *93*: 25–33, 1999.

116. Balabanian, K., B. Lagane, S. Infantino, K.Y. Chow, J. Harriague, B. Moepps, F. Arenzana-Seisdedos, M. Thelen, and F. Bachelerie. The chemokine SDF-1/CXCL12 binds to and signals through the orphan receptor RDC1 in T lymphocytes. J Biol Chem *280*: 35760–6, 2005.

117. Burns, J.M., B.C. Summers, Y. Wang, A. Melikian, R. Berahovich, Z. Miao, M.E. Penfold, M.J. Sunshine, D.R. Littman, C.J. Kuo, K. Wei, B.E. McMaster, K. Wright, M.C. Howard, and T.J. Schall. A novel chemokine receptor for SDF-1 and I-TAC involved in cell survival, cell adhesion, and tumor development. J Exp Med *203*: 2201–13, 2006.

118. Miao, Z., K.E. Luker, B.C. Summers, R. Berahovich, M.S. Bhojani, A. Rehemtulla, C.G. Kleer, J.J. Essner, A. Nasevicius, G.D. Luker, M.C. Howard, and T.J. Schall. CXCR7 (RDC1) promotes breast and lung tumor growth in vivo and is expressed on tumor-associated vasculature. Proc Natl Acad Sci U S A *104*: 15735–40, 2007.

119. Wang, J., Y. Shiozawa, Y. Wang, Y. Jung, K.J. Pienta, R. Mehra, R. Loberg, and R.S. Taichman. The Role of CXCR7/RDC1 as a Chemokine Receptor for CXCL12/SDF-1 in Prostate Cancer. J Biol Chem *283*: 4283–94, 2008.

120. Dambly-Chaudiere, C., N. Cubedo, and A. Ghysen. Control of cell migration in the development of the posterior lateral line: antagonistic interactions between the chemokine receptors CXCR4 and CXCR7/RDC1. BMC Dev Biol *7*: 23, 2007.

121. Arenberg, D.A., S.L. Kunkel, P.J. Polverini, S.B. Morris, M.D. Burdick, M.C. Glass, D.T. Taub, M.D. Iannettoni, R.I. Whyte, and R.M. Strieter. Interferon-gamma-inducible protein 10 (IP-10) is an angiostatic factor that inhibits human non-small cell lung cancer (NSCLC) tumorigenesis and spontaneous metastases. J Exp Med *184*: 981–92, 1996.

122. Minna, J.D. "Neoplasms if the lung," in *Principles of Internal Medicine*, ed. Isselbacher, K.J. (New York: McGraew-Hill, 1991).

123. Carney, D.N. "Cancers of the lungs," in *Pulmonary Diseases and Disorders*, ed. Fishman, A.P. (New York: McGraw-Hill, 1988).

124. Yuan, A., Y. Pan-Chyr, Y. Chong-Jen, Y. Lee, Y. Yu-Tuang, C. Chi-Long, L. Lee, K. Sow-Hsong, and L. Kwen-Tay. Tumor angiogenesis correlates with histologic type and metastasis in non-small cell lung cancer. Am J Resp Crit Care Med *152*: 2157–62, 1995.

125. Feldman, A.L., J. Friedl, T.E. Lans, S.K. Libutti, D. Lorang, M.S. Miller, E.M. Turner, S.M. Hewitt, and H.R. Alexander. Retroviral gene transfer of interferon-inducible protein 10 inhibits growth of human melanoma xenografts. Int J Cancer *99*: 149–53, 2002.

126. Addison, C.L., D.A. Arenberg, S.B. Morris, Y.Y. Xue, M.D. Burdick, M.S. Mulligan, M.D. Iannettoni, and R.M. Strieter. The CXC chemokine, monokine induced by interferon-gamma, inhibits non-small cell lung carcinoma tumor growth and metastasis. Hum Gene Ther *11*: 247–61, 2000.

127. Gurtsevitch, V.E., G.T. O'Conor, and G.M. Lenoir. Burkitt's lymphoma cell lines reveal different degrees of tumorigenicity in nude mice. Int J Cancer *41*: 87–95, 1988.

128. Sgadari, C., A.L. Angiolillo, B.W. Cherney, S.E. Pike, J.M. Farber, L.G. Koniaris, P. Vanguri, P.R. Burd, N. Sheikh, G. Gupta, J. Teruya-Feldstein, and G. Tosato. Interferon-inducible protein-10 identified as a mediator of tumor necrosis in vivo. Proc. Natl. Acad. Sci. U S A *93*: 13791–6, 1996.

129. Sgadari, C., J.M. Farber, A.L. Angiolillo, F. Liao, J. Teruya-Feldstein, P.R. Burd, L. Yao, G. Gupta, C. Kanegane, and G. Tosato. Mig, the monokine induced by interferon-gamma, promotes tumor necrosis in vivo. Blood *89*: 2635–43, 1997.

130. Sgadari, C., A.L. Angiolillo, and G. Tosato. Inhibition of angiogenesis by interleukin-12 is mediated by the interferon-inducible protein 10. Blood *87*: 3877–82, 1996.

131. Teruya-Feldstein, J., E.S. Jaffe, P.R. Burd, H. Kanegane, D.W. Kingma, W.H. Wilson, D.L. Longo, and G. Tosato. The role of Mig, the monokine induced by interferon-gamma, and IP-10, the interferon-gamma-inducible protein-10, in tissue necrosis and vascular damage associated with Epstein-Barr virus-positive lymphoproliferative disease. Blood *90*: 4099–105, 1997.

132. Moser, M. Regulation of Th1/Th2 development by antigen-presenting cells in vivo. Immunobiology *204*: 551–7, 2001.

133. Sharma, S., S.C. Yang, S. Hillinger, L.X. Zhu, M. Huang, R.K. Batra, J.F. Lin, M.D. Burdick, R.M. Strieter, and S.M. Dubinett. SLC/CCL21-mediated anti-tumor responses require IFNgamma, MIG/CXCL9 and IP-10/CXCL10. Mol Cancer *2*: 22, 2003.

134. Sharma, S., M. Stolina, J. Luo, R.M. Strieter, M. Burdick, L.X. Zhu, R.K. Batra, and S.M. Dubinett. Secondary lymphoid tissue chemokine mediates T cell-dependent anti-tumor responses in vivo. J Immunol *164*: 4558–63, 2000.

135. Tannenbaum, C.S., R. Tubbs, D. Armstrong, J.H. Finke, R.M. Bukowski, and T.A. Hamilton. The CXC chemokines IP-10 and Mig are necessary for IL-12-mediated regression of the mouse RENCA tumor. J Immunol *161*: 927–32, 1998.

136. Pan, J., M.D. Burdick, J.A. Belperio, Y.Y. Xue, C. Gerard, S. Sharma, S.M. Dubinett, and R.M. Strieter. CXCR3/CXCR3 ligand biological axis impairs RENCA tumor growth by a mechanism of immunoangiostasis. J Immunol *176*: 1456–64, 2006.

The Roles of Chemokines and Chemokine Receptors in Prostate Cancer

Thorsten Eismann, Nadine Huber, and Alex B. Lentsch

Abstract Cancer of the prostate is the second most diagnosed cancer in men. The pathogenesis of this disease is complex, but is known to involve multiple factors that affect tumor growth, invasion, and metastasis. One group of such factors are CXC chemokines, which are a subset of chemotactic cytokines which, through their receptors, have angiogenic or angiostatic properties. This review will discuss our current understanding of the various functional roles that CXC chemokines and their receptors play in the development and progression of prostate cancer.

Introduction

Prostate cancer is the second most frequently diagnosed cancer in men, with 782 600 new cases projected to occur in 2007 [31]. Incidence rates vary widely between countries and ethnic populations, and disease rates differ by more that 100-fold between populations. The lowest yearly incidence rates occur in Asia (1.9 cases per 100 000 in Tainjin, China) and the highest in North America and Scandinavia, especially in African-Americans (272 cases per 100 000) [79, 80]. African-American men have furthermore the highest mortality rate for prostate cancer of any racial or ethnic group in the US. The age-adjusted prostate cancer-related mortality is 2.4 times higher for African-Americans than for whites. This difference accounts for about 40% of the overall cancer mortality disparity between African-American and white men [31].

The pathogenesis of prostate cancer reflects both hereditary and environmental components, and growing evidence suggests a role for chronic inflammation in prostate cancer [21, 22, 78]. The exact mechanisms by which inflammatory processes contribute to the initiation and progression of prostate cancer remain

A.B. Lentsch (✉)
Department of Surgery, University of Cincinnati College of Medicine, Cincinnati, OH 45267-0558, USA
e-mail: alex.lentsch@uc.edu

A.M. Fulton (ed.), *Chemokine Receptors in Cancer*, Cancer Drug Discovery and Development, DOI 10.1007/978-1-60327-267-4_9,
© Humana Press, a part of Springer Science+Business Media, LLC 2009

elusive. Inflammation-associated DNA damage, proliferation, angiogenesis, invasion, and metastasis may all play a role in the development and progression of prostate cancer [5, 17, 67, 68].

It is well established that chemokines play a critical role in inflammation and immunity. Interactions between chemokines and their receptors are essential for the inflammatory pathway, but it is now appreciated that the chemokine receptor system can be altered dramatically in neoplastic tissue. Moreover, chemokines induce direct effects on stromal and prostate cancer cells in addition to their roles in regulating leukocyte recruitment.

Human chemokines, encoded by 43 genes, are a family of structurally related and mainly secreted molecules, defined by a tetra-cysteine motif. Depending on the motif displayed by the first two cysteines, they have been classified into CXC (or alpha), CC (beta), C (gamma), and CX_3C (delta) chemokines (where X is any amino acid) [83, 108]. Chemokines can also be classified according to their production condition into pro-inflammatory (that is, produced in response to inflammatory or immunological stimuli (such as CCL2, CCL5, and CXCL8) or homeostatic (that is, produced constitutively, such as CXCL12, CXCL13, CXCL14, and CCL19) chemokines [54]. Chemokines bind to a subfamily of seven-transmembrane G-protein-coupled receptors, which at present include 18 human chemokine receptors, to induce direct cell migration. They are classified as CCR, CXCR, CX_3CR, and XCR on the basis of the class of chemokines they are able to bind [65]. In addition, the discovery of atypical receptors with high structural homology to other chemokine receptors has strengthened the proposal that the genome contains specialized receptors to regulate the chemokine network. These decoy receptors are able to recognize certain inflammatory cytokines with a high affinity and specificity, but are structurally incapable of signaling or presenting the agonist to signal receptor complexes [55]. The subfamily of decoy receptors includes Duffy antigen receptor for chemokines (DARC) [39], D6 (also known as CCBP2) [9, 73] and CCX-CKR (also known as CCRL1) [33]. Detailed structure-function analyses of this receptor subfamily have not yet been accomplished. It is known, however, that structural determinants that are required for ligand-induced signaling, such as the key residues in the second intracellular loop near the conserved DRY (Asp-Arg-Tyr) motif, which is involved in coupling G proteins, are not conserved in these receptors. The DRYLAIV motif is altered to DKYLEIV in D6 [73] whereas DARC apparently lacks canonical intracellular signaling motifs [15] and does not support any detectable ligand-induced signaling or direct cell migration [70].

Role of Chemokines and Their Receptors in Prostate Cancer Angiogenesis and Tumor Growth

Angiogenesis is the process of new blood vessel growth and is a critical biological process under both physiologic and pathologic conditions. For purposes of this discussion, angiogenesis and neovascularization will be used interchangeably in the context of pathologic (tumorigenesis) or aberrant angiogenesis (chronic inflammation/fibroproliferative disorders). Immunohistochemical techniques have shown that microvessel density is increased in prostate cancer specimens, compared with benign prostate tissue, and that vessel density is an independent predictor of pathologic stage in patients with prostate cancer [7, 10, 106]. CXC chemokines display disparate roles in the regulation of angiogenesis and tumor growth. CXC chemokines have been shown to exert either angiogenic or angiostatic activities depending on the presence or absence of the amino acid sequence Glu-Leu-Arg (ELR motif). The ELR motif, which is found in the amino terminus of all angiogenic CXC chemokines but in none of the angiostatic CXC chemokines, has been shown to be required for angiogenic activity by site-directed mutagenesis studies [94]. Table 1 shows CXC chemokines with angiogenic and angiostatic properties, as well as the receptors to which they bind.

Angiogenic CXC chemokines have been implicated in the pathogenesis of prostate cancer [27, 40, 42, 45, 46, 48, 62, 64, 76, 82, 90, 100, 101]. Immunohistochemical studies of human prostate tissues have shown that prostate cancer cells express abundant amounts of CXCL8 whereas normal prostate and benign prostatic hyperplasia tissue express very little, if any, CXCL8 [27]. In addition, other studies have shown that serum levels of CXCL8 are not increased in patients with benign prostatic hyperplasia, but are greatly increased in patients with prostate cancer [48, 101]. Additionally, increased mRNA expression of CXCL8 was associated with both the Gleason score and even stronger with the pathologic stage of prostate cancer [100]. These clinical findings are supported by in vitro studies of prostate cancer cell lines. A number of prostate cancer cell lines produce high levels of angiogenic CXC chemokines endogenously and stimulation with cytokines induces even greater production of these mediators

Table 1 CXC chemokines with angiogenic and angiostatic activities including their receptors that bind the angiogenic and angiostatic CXC chemokines

Angiogenic CXC chemokines (ELR$^+$)			Angiostatic CXC chemokines (ELR$^-$)		
Current nomenclature	Old nomenclature	Receptor(s)	Current nomenclature	Old nomenclature	Receptor(s)
CXCL1	GROα	CXCR1, CXCR2, DARC	CXCL4	PF4	CXCR3
CXCL2	GROβ	CXCR2, DARC	CXCL9	MIG	CXCR3
CXCL3	GROγ	CXCR2, DARC	CXCL10	IP-10	CXCR3
CXCL5	ENA-78	CXCR2	CXCL11	I-TAC	CXCR3
CXCL6	GCP-2	CXCR1, CXCR2	CXCL12	SDF-1	CXCR4
CXCL7	NAP-2	CXCR2, DARC	CXCL14	BRAK	Unknown
CXCL8	IL-8	CXCR1, CXCR2, DARC			

[27, 62, 90. 101]. It was demonstrated that endogenous CXCL8 from human prostate cancer cells is able to modulate the expression of several genes that are involved in regulating metastasis, suggesting not only an influence in angiogenesis, but also in invasion/metastasis [45]. Furthermore, when prostate cancer cells were injected into severe combined immune deficient (SCID) mice, tumor growth could be attenuated with blocking antibodies to CXCL1 or CXCL8 [62]. Studies from our laboratory have shown that prostate cancer cells in mice express higher levels of angiogenic chemokines than normal prostate tissues [90]. Combined, these studies suggest that ELR^+CXC chemokines function to promote neovascularization in prostate cancer.

Much less is known regarding the mechanisms contributing to increased microvessel density in prostate carcinoma. The complex milieu of tumor stroma interactions probably requires several factors that are involved in different aspects of the angiogenic process. Our laboratory has shown that normal prostate epithelial cells produce relatively high amounts of angiostatic CXC chemokines and low amounts of angiogenic CXC chemokines [90]. It could be proposed that this balance of angiogenic/angiostatic CXC chemokines maintains a homeostatic milieu. Cells derived from primary prostate cancer had reduced production of angiostatic CXC chemokines and greatly increased production of angiogenic CXC chemokines. Cells derived from metastatic prostate cancer had even less production of angiostatic CXC chemokines and far greater production of angiogenic CXC chemokines. Normal prostate epithelial cell production of angiostatic CXC chemokines was linked to activation of the transcription factor, signal transducer and activator of transcription (STAT) 1. STAT1 has been shown to induce the angiostatic CXC chemokines CXCL9 and CXCL10 [30]. Further, the activation of STAT1 is implicated in shaping antitumor immune responses [89]. In prostate cancer cells, STAT1 activation was reduced, consistent with the reduced production of angiostatic chemokines [90]. It was also determined that increased production of angiogenic CXC chemokines in prostate cancer cells was due to progressive activation of nuclear factor (NF)-κB [90]. Constitutive activation of NF-κB in prostate cancer cells has previously been demonstrated [32, 74, 95]. More recently it was suggested that NF-κB is responsible for the upregulation of CXCR1 and CXCR2 expression in hypoxic prostate cancer cells, contributing to a survival advantage in these cells [58]. In prostate cancer significant areas of hypoxia could be detected, and greater hypoxia scores are associated with more aggressive prostate cancer [12, 63]. Prostate cancer cells seem to respond to hypoxia by regulating the transcription and increasing the expression of angiogenic factors, such as ELR^+CXC chemokines that act upon endothelial cells to promote new blood vessel formation to promote cell survival and tumor growth.

There is abundant evidence that the receptor CXCR2 regulates the angiogenic process in a number of model systems. Gene knockout or antibody blockade of CXCR2 prevented CXC chemokine-mediated angiogenesis in a corneal micropocket assay [2]. Subsequently, it was shown that blockade of CXCR2 function disrupted endothelial cell chemotaxis and tube formation induced by CXCL8 [36]. In prostate cancer, the expression of CXCR2 is correlated with cell proliferation and microvessel density [64]. Our laboratory has recently demonstrated that mice lacking the gene for CXCR2 show significant smaller prostate cancers than their wild-type counterparts. These findings were associated with reduced angiogenesis as well as decreased expression of matrix metalloproteinases in prostate cancers of CXCR2-knockout mice [91, 92]. In human prostate cancer, CXCR2 has been shown to be exclusively expressed in the neuroendocrine cells [40]. Interestingly, the same study revealed that CXCR1 was overexpressed in the luminal malignant secretory cells. Although the CXCL8 receptor CXCR1 is rarely expressed in benign epithelial cells, its expression is increased in prostate intraepithelial neoplasia (PIN) and further increased in invasive tumors [64], suggesting a paracrine mechanism whereby CXCL8 produced by the neuroendocrine prostate cancer cells may promote the proliferation of the non-neuroendocrine prostate cancer cells in the absence of androgen. The contribution of the ELR$^+$ chemokine CXCL8 in androgen-independent growth and progression of prostate cancer is supported by a recent study, suggesting that CXCL8-induced growth is mediated by CXCR1 [4].

Other studies have shown that the receptor CXCR3 might also play a role in the regulation of prostate tumor growth [66, 91, 92]. It was suggested that overexpression of the ELR$^-$ chemokine CXCL10 in prostate cancer cells causes a significant increase in its CXCR3 expression, resulting in inhibition of cell proliferation [66]. Our laboratory further demonstrated that conditioned media from normal prostate epithelial cells actually decreased endothelial cell chemotaxis below that of media alone, whereas conditioned media from prostate cancer cells showed an increase in endothelial cell chemotaxis [91, 92]. These findings imply that secretions by normal prostate epithelial cells would not be expected to stimulate angiogenesis and tumor growth. In the same system, when two prominent CXCR3 ligands (CXCL10 and CXCL11) were neutralized, the conditioned media had a higher chemotactic response toward endothelial cells, suggesting that malignant transformation of prostate epithelial cells may turn off production of ELR$^-$ CXC chemokines and this may contribute to a pro-angiogenic milieu. This concept was confirmed with studies of CXCR3-knockout mice. In these mice, prostate carcinomas could be detected at a much earlier age and had increased neovascularization when compared to wild-type controls [91, 92].

Role of Chemokines and Their Receptors in Prostate Cancer Invasion and Metastasis

Besides the role of chemokines and their receptors in angiogenesis, they also seem to be involved in the process of tumor cell migration, invasion, and metastasis. It is known that certain tumors exhibit specific patterns of metastasis to, or invasion in, certain organs. In other words, tumor cells do not migrate randomly. Metastasis is a multistep process in which tumor cells gain access to the vasculature in the primary tumor, survive the circulation, arrest in the microvasculature of the target organ, exit from the microvasculature, and proliferate in the target tissues. It has been shown that greater numbers of tumor vessels increase the opportunity for tumor cells to enter the circulation [49, 50]. As for prostate carcinoma, a histological analysis has shown that there is a significant correlation between the density of microvessels of invasive prostate carcinoma and the incidence of metastases [106]. However, the specific migration of cancer cells, which is recognized as a critical step in metastasis, is a phenomenon that may be determined by the chemokine receptors they express and by the chemokines expressed in the target organs. There is some evidence supporting this hypothesis. It has been reported that different human prostate cancer cell lines from the same general cancer type use distinct angiogenic CXC chemokines [62]. Since prostate cancer has the tendency to metastasize to bone, there has been some focus on bone-associated chemokines and cancer cell surface-associated chemokine receptor function in prostate cancer cells. Recent reports indicate that the CXCL12/CXCR4 chemokine axis is involved in prostate cancer metastasis [61, 98, 99]. Cell surface expression of CXCR4 in prostate cancer cells has been implicated in "homing" to microenvironments of high CXCL12 chemokine concentrations [98, 99], such as in bone marrow [77]. During this process, the circulating cancer cell mimics hematopoetic and immune cells in terms of localizing to high CXCL12-expressing sites, firm adhesion to endothelial cells, transmigration across the blood vessel wall, and migration toward the chemokine source; a process that was recently suggested to occur also in prostate cancer bone metastasis [96]. Moreover it was demonstrated that CXCL12 and CXCR4 are key elements in the growth of metastatic prostate cancer [102, 103].

In prostate cancer, it has been reported that androgen receptor negatively regulates CXCR4 [3], which leads to the suggestion that loss of androgen receptor enhances prostate cancer migration. This may be important to the development of metastasis because as prostate cancer progresses, androgen receptor expression is altered. Another mechanism through which CXCR4 could be regulated and promote metastasis, could be through NF-κB-mediated induction of CXCR4. NF-κB has been shown to upregulate chemotaxis by inducing CXCR4 expression in breast cancer cells [37]. However, inhibition of CXCR4 in vivo only partially blocks the metastatic behavior of prostate cancer, suggesting that other factors play a role in the control of tissue-specific migration [97]. A recent report indicates that the receptor CXCR7 has also a function as a chemokine receptor for CXCL12. In vitro and in vivo studies with prostate cancer cells suggest that alterations in CXCR7 expression are associated with enhanced adhesive and invasive activities in addition to a survival advantage [102, 103]. In addition, it was shown that CXCR7 also regulates the expression of the pro-angiogenic factors CXCL8 or VEGF, suggesting a role in the regulation of tumor angiogenesis. Furthermore, it was demonstrated that signaling through or expression of CXCR4 alters CXCR7 levels, while CXCR7 expression is not directly linked to CXCR4 expression [102, 103]. CXCR7 was shown to form functional heterodimers with CXCR4 that potentiated CXCL12 signaling [93]. A previous report supports the role of CXCR7 in having an affect on a spectrum of important biological and pathological processes, including cell growth/survival and adhesion, as well as the promotion of tumor growth [11]. However, it was suggested that the CXCR7 signaling pathway might be distinct from the typical G-protein-coupled receptor mechanism.

Role of Decoy Receptors in Prostate Cancer

As mentioned earlier, the biological activities of chemokines are mediated by distinct members of the rhodopsin-like seven-transmembrane domain, G-protein-coupled receptor superfamily [65]. Other receptors exist that bind chemokines with high affinity and specificity [16]. However, these receptors are structurally incapable of transducing signals and are therefore designated as decoy receptors.

Pro-inflammatory CC chemokines control inflammatory leukocyte recruitment and behavior by signaling through the receptors CCR1-5. Many of these same chemokines also bind to the decoy receptor D6 (see Table 2). In vitro biochemical investigations have revealed that D6 appears to be specialized for the rapid and continuous internalization and degradation of its ligands [8, 29, 105]. Further, it was demonstrated that D6 reduces the bioavailability of pro-inflammatory chemokines in vivo to ensure appropriate resolution of inflammatory responses [43, 56, 57, 107]. A recent report showed that D6-deficient mice have increased susceptibility to cutaneous tumor development in response to a tumor-promoting agent and that D6 deletion is sufficient to make resistant mouse strains susceptible to invasive squamous cell carcinoma [72]. This tumor susceptibility directly correlated with the extent of T-cell and mast-cell recruitment, cell types known to support the development of skin

Table 2 The atypical chemokine receptor family

Atypical receptor	Other name(s)	Chemokine ligands	Signaling receptor(s) potentially regulated
D6	ccbp2	CCL2, CCL3, hCCL3L1, CCL4, hCCL4L1, CCL5, CCL7, CCL8, CCL11, CCL12, CCL13, CCL14, CCL17, CCL22	CCR1, CCR2, CCR3, CCR4, CCR5
DARC	ccbp3	CCL2, CCL5, CCL11, CCL13, CCL14, CCL17, CXCL1, CXCL2, CXCL3, hCXCL7, hCXCL8	CCR1, CCR2, CCR3, CCR4, CCR5, CXCR1, CXCR2
CCX-CKR	CCR11, CCRl1, ccbp1	CCL19, CCL21, CCL25, hCXCL13	CCR7, CCR9, hCXCR5

tumors in mice [13, 26]. These data suggest an important role of the pro-inflammatory CC chemokine network in the early stages of a progressive, multistep de novo tumorigenesis, where D6-mediated chemokine sequestration may be a novel and effective method of tumor suppression. It will be interesting to determine the nature of the involvement of D6 in human tumorigenesis, which may be of relevance to those tumors in which inflammation has been directly implicated in the tumorigenic process, as is postulated for prostate cancer [35]. CCL2, a member of the cytokine/chemokine superfamily, is a ligand for CCR2 as well as for D6 and is known to promote the migration of monocytes and macrophages to sites of inflammation. CCL2 expression was shown to correlate with advanced stages of prostate cancer and that prostate cancer cells produced CCL2 in vitro [52]. A recent study suggests a contribution of CCL2 to prostate cancer growth through the regulation of macrophage infiltration and enhanced angiogenesis within the tumor [51]. It is tempting to speculate that chemokine sequestration by D6 might be involved in the tumorigenesis of prostate cancer and that the nature of the inflammatory infiltrate might determine its pro- or antitumorigenic tendencies. However, there is no direct evidence in prostate cancer thus far to test these hypotheses.

The DARC is a decoy receptor that is highly associated with prostate carninoma and is expressed primarily on erythrocytes and vascular endothelial cells [34]. It was originally identified as an erythroid receptor for *Plasmodium vivax* [60] and was subsequently shown to have a chemokine-binding capacity [39, 69]. More than 95% of Africans in the endemic regions and approximately 70% of African-Americans lack erythroid expression of the DARC, as a natural selection against *P. vivax* infections [59]. However, these individuals retain DARC expression on their vascular endothelium [75]. The DARC is associated with caveolae vesicles in endothelial cells, and these structures are commonly associated with transcellular transport of their cargo [14], leading to the hypothesis that the DARC is involved in the transcytosis, or neutralization of chemokines at endothelial barriers [47]. Additional evidence for a functional role of the DARC has emerged from studies on mice lacking the expression of DARC on both erythrocytes and endothelial cells [20, 53], proposing that the DARC on erythrocytes could possibly function to inactivate circulating chemokines by acting as a "sink", removing excess chemokines from the bloodstream [19]. Work from our laboratory supports this theory that the DARC is capable of binding and clearing chemokines from sites of overproduction, such as inflammatory foci and act therefore as a biological sink for chemokines [20]. In situ ligand-binding assays have demonstrated that radiolabeled chemokines selectively bind to venular endothelial cells and assessment of ligand cross-competition provided a fingerprint of chemokine-binding specificity of venular endothelial cells identical to that of the DARC [41, 87]. Indeed, studies using DARC-knockout mice have shown that this endothelial cell-chemokine binding is DARC dependent [71]. In vitro studies revealed that endothelial DARC might play a role in the transport of chemokines across the endothelial barrier to maintain tissue chemokine gradients [47].

The DARC also appears to have a regulatory role in angiogenesis. Transgenic mice overexpressing the DARC on the vascular endothelium display a reduced angiogenic response to the angiogenic (ELR^+) murine CXC chemokine, MIP-2, in the corneal micropocket assay [24]. These studies suggest that the DARC may sequester chemokines, preventing them from activating CXCR2 on endothelial cells, and therefore blocking angiogenic signals from this receptor. Other reports further demonstrate that overexpressing the DARC in endothelial or tumor cells reduces angiogenesis, supporting the scavenging effects of the DARC on angiogenic CXC chemokines [1, 24]. Recent studies from our laboratory demonstrate that mice lacking the DARC have higher concentrations of ELR^+ CXC chemokines in prostate tumors than wild-type mice, in addition to increased angiogenesis and tumor growth [91, 92]. These findings suggest that erythrocyte DARC functions as a sponge for angiogenic chemokines. This hypothesis is illustrated in Fig. 1. As blood flows through the tumor microcirculation, DARC on erythrocytes binds and removes angiogenic chemokines. Based on this hypothesis, the lack of erythrocyte expression of DARC, as occurs in approximately 70% of the African-American population, may remove one of the supporting mechanisms to restrict tumor growth. Individuals lacking erythrocyte expression of DARC would have higher intratumor concentrations of ELR^+ CXC chemokines, resulting in increased tumor angiogenesis and growth. Thus, lack of DARC expression on erythrocytes may predispose men of African descent to more aggressive prostate cancer growth.

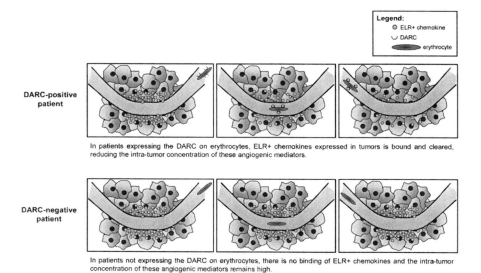

Legend:
- ⊙ ELR+ chemokine
- ∪ DARC
- ⬤ erythrocyte

DARC-positive patient

In patients expressing the DARC on erythrocytes, ELR+ chemokines expressed in tumors is bound and cleared, reducing the intra-tumor concentration of these angiogenic mediators.

DARC-negative patient

In patients not expressing the DARC on erythrocytes, there is no binding of ELR+ chemokines and the intra-tumor concentration of these angiogenic mediators remains high.

Fig. 1 Model of erythrocyte DARC function in the prostate cancer microenvironment. Expression of erythrocyte DARC binds and clears angiogenic ELR^+CXC chemokines from the tumor. However, lack of the erythrocyte DARC results in a higher than normal intratumor concentration of angiogenic chemokines

Therefore, early screening of this population for erythrocyte DARC expression may be predictive of the aggressiveness of prostate cancer growth.

A recent study has also suggested that DARC may prevent prostate cancer cell proliferation, through interaction with the tetraspanin cell surface protein known as the leukocyte cell surface marker CD82, or KAI1 [6]. In this study, a yeast two-hybrid screen identified DARC as a binding partner to CD82, which is expressed on the surface of prostate cancer cells. This interaction led to decreased proliferation, induction of senescence, and decreased metastasis [6]. An investigation of murine melanoma tumor growth indicated that endothelial cell overexpression of DARC reduced the growth of blood vessels in the tumor and the tumor growth rate, whereas endothelial cell overexpression of CXCR2 had the reverse effect on neovascularization and tumor growth [38]. The lymphocyte density as well as the number of macrophages in the tumors from DARC-transgenic mice was shown to be significantly higher than in either the tumors from wild-type or CXCR2-transgenic mice [38]. This is in accordance with a study suggesting a survival advantage for patients with tumors containing high numbers of tumor-infiltrating lymphocytes [88]. Thus, it is possible that the DARC may possibly capture chemotactic chemokines at the basolateral surface of the endothelial cells, internalize them, and transport them to the apical or luminal surface of the endothelial cells. In this manner, leukocytes flowing in the blood stream adhere to the endothelial cell in an integrin-dependent process and extravasate through the endothelium to underlying tissue where they migrate along a chemokine gradient to the target site. In addition to the regulation of angiogenic chemokine levels in the prostate cancer microenvironment, the DARC may also limit tumor growth and metastasis through other mechanisms, since there is growing evidence that the DARC is able to regulate the biological effects of chemokines in three distinct ways, either through scavenging, retention, or transport.

Future Perspective

The presence of pro-inflammatory chemokines may not be beneficial in a chronic inflammatory disease, but may be desirable in diseases where the immune response needs to be promoted, such as cancer. In theory, any chemokine capable of inducing the migration of T cells, dendritic cells, and/or macrophages could promote the regression of a tumor mass by boosting the immune response against the tumor. Current therapeutic approaches revealed only a modest impact on survival outcomes for patients with advanced prostate cancer. Recent progress in the identification of tumor-associated antigens and derived T-cell epitopes paved the way for the design of novel T-cell or antibody-based strategies in patients with prostate cancer [44]. T-cell-based immunotherapy of tumors has emerged with the observation that $CD8^+$ cytotoxic T cells (CTLs) provide a high capability to recognize and destroy tumor cells that expose peptides derived from tumor-associated antigens in the complex with human leukocyte antigen (HLA) class I molecules [85]. Some clinical studies have focused on the adoptive transfer of cytotoxic effector cells. In prostate cancer, most of the targets for T-cell-mediated immunotherapy revealed tumor regression in cancer patients [25]. CD4$^+$ T cells also play an important role in antitumor immunity since they recognize peptides in the context of HLA class II molecules [104]. Several studies have demonstrated that CD40–CD40 ligand interactions between DCs and CD4$^+$ T cells activate dendritic cells for effective priming and activation. Furthermore CD4$^+$ T cells are essential in the maintenance of CD8$^+$ T-cell effector functions by secreting cytokines, such as interleukin-2, that are required for CD8$^+$ T-cell growth and proliferation, and they can eradicate tumor cells directly. In prostate cancer most of the targets for T-cell-mediated immunotherapy are differentiation antigens that are specifically expressed by normal and malignant prostate tissue [44]. Prostate cancer is also an attractive target for antibody-based therapies because the nonvital function of the prostate extends the spectrum of potential target molecules by tissue-specific markers not restricted to tumor, and the usually small size of metastases is beneficial for antibody access and penetration [86]. The clinical efficiency, however, of the different immunotherapeutic strategies, which represent safe and feasible concepts, is still limited for the majority of patients with advanced prostate cancer, owing to various immune evasion mechanisms mediated by tumors [23, 81].

Another therapeutic approach to limit prostate cancer growth is reducing tumor angiogenesis. Today several anti-angiogenic drugs are already being tested in clinical trials. One of these is thalidomide. Investigators examined the clinical activity of this anti-angiogenic drug, initially as a monotherapy in patients with androgen-independent prostate cancer, demonstrating in 18% of patients a greater than 50% decrease in their PSA levels [28]. When treated with a combined therapy of docetaxel (a well-established antimitotic chemotherapy medication) and thalidomide, half the patients showed a 50% decrease in PSA levels, compared to 37% of those treated with docetaxel alone [18]. However, only 26% of patients with hormone refractory, metastatic prostate cancer that were treated with combined therapy of thalidomide and dexamethasone after chemotherapy have a greater than 50% PSA reduction with no radiologic progression [84]. Those clinical trials are in their early stages and larger randomized trials are needed to better evaluate the efficacy of this and similar regimens in patients with advanced prostate cancer.

Conclusion

During malignant transformation of prostate epithelial cells, reprogramming of the transcriptional machinery occurs and these cells begin to produce high amounts of ELR$^+$CXC chemokines. These chemokines bind to their receptor, CXCR2, on vascular endothelial cells and promote neovascular formation by

enhancing endothelial cell chemotaxis toward the tumor cells and tube formation. In prostate cancer, DARC appears to function as a molecular mop by
reducing intratumor concentrations of angiogenic chemokines. Thus, a genetic
alteration in men of African ancestry may contribute to enhanced tumor
growth and increased angiogenesis as a result of higher intratumor concentrations of ELR $^+$ chemokines. Additionally, DARC expressed on endothelial cells
may also function as a shuttling molecule for chemokines and might play a role
in chemokine-mediated leukocyte recruitment.

Even as new approaches to treat patients with prostate cancer show promise,
further improvements must still be made. Targeting chemokine-mediated processes along with stimulation of an enhanced immune response may yield
important new advances in therapy. Other such combinatorial therapies must
be explored if we are to make inroads in the treatment of patients with advanced
stages of this disease.

References

1. Addison, C. L., J. A. Belperio, M. D. Burdick and R. M. Strieter (2004). "Overexpression
   of the duffy antigen receptor for chemokines (DARC) by NSCLC tumor cells results in
   increased tumor necrosis." *BMC Cancer* **4**: 28.
2. Addison, C. L., T. O. Daniel, M. D. Burdick, H. Liu, J. E. Ehlert, Y. Y. Xue, L. Buechi, A.
   Walz, A. Richmond and R. M. Strieter (2000). "The CXC chemokine receptor 2, CXCR2,
   is the putative receptor for ELR+ CXC chemokine-induced angiogenic activity."
   J Immunol **165**(9): 5269–5277.
3. Akashi, T., K. Koizumi, O. Nagakawa, H. Fuse and I. Saiki (2006). "Androgen receptor
   negatively influences the expression of chemokine receptors (CXCR4, CCR1) and ligand-
   mediated migration in prostate cancer DU-145." *Oncol Rep* **16** (4): 831–836.
4. Araki, S., Y. Omori, D. Lyn, R. K. Singh, D. M. Meinbach, Y. Sandman, V. B. Lokeshwar
   and B. L. Lokeshwar (2007). "Interleukin-8 is a molecular determinant of androgen
   independence and progression in prostate cancer." *Cancer Res* **67** (14): 6854–6862.
5. Balkwill, F. and A. Mantovani (2001). "Inflammation and cancer: back to Virchow?"
   Lancet **357** (9255): 539–545.
6. Bandyopadhyay, S., R. Zhan, A. Chaudhuri, M. Watabe, S. K. Pai, S. Hirota, S. Hosobe, T.
   Tsukada, K. Miura, Y. Takano, K. Saito, M. E. Pauza, S. Hayashi, Y. Wang, S. Mohinta, T.
   Mashimo, M. Iiizumi, E. Furuta and K. Watabe (2006). "Interaction of KAI1 on tumor cells
   with DARC on vascular endothelium leads to metastasis suppression." *Nat Med* **12** (8):
   933–938.
7. Bigler, S. A., R. E. Deering and M. K. Brawer (1993). "Comparison of microscopic
   vascularity in benign and malignant prostate tissue." *Hum Pathol* **24** (2): 220–226.
8. Bonecchi, R., M. Locati, E. Galliera, M. Vulcano, M. Sironi, A. M. Fra, M. Gobbi,
   A. Vecchi, S. Sozzani, B. Haribabu, J. Van Damme and A. Mantovani (2004). "Differential
   recognition and scavenging of native and truncated macrophage-derived chemokine
   (macrophage-derived chemokine/CC chemokine ligand 22) by the D6 decoy receptor."
   J Immunol **172** (8): 4972–4976.
9. Bonini, J. A., S. K. Martin, F. Dralyuk, M. W. Roe, L. H. Philipson and D. F. Steiner
   (1997). "Cloning, expression, and chromosomal mapping of a novel human CC-chemokine
   receptor (CCR10) that displays high-affinity binding for MCP-1 and MCP-3." *DNA Cell
   Biol* **16** (10): 1249–1256.

10. Brawer, M. K., R. E. Deering, M. Brown, S. D. Preston and S. A. Bigler (1994). "Predictors of pathologic stage in prostatic carcinoma. The role of neovascularity." *Cancer* **73** (3): 678–687.

11. Burns, J. M., B. C. Summers, Y. Wang, A. Melikian, R. Berahovich, Z. Miao, M. E. Penfold, M. J. Sunshine, D. R. Littman, C. J. Kuo, K. Wei, B. E. McMaster, K. Wright, M. C. Howard and T. J. Schall (2006). " A novel chemokine receptor for SDF-1 and I-TAC involved in cell survival, cell adhesion, and tumor development." *J Exp Med* **203** (9): 2201–2213.

12. Carnell, D. M., R. E. Smith, F. M. Daley, M. I. Saunders, S. M. Bentzen and P. J. Hoskin (2006). "An immunohistochemical assessment of hypoxia in prostate carcinoma using pimonidazole: implications for radioresistance." *Int J Radiat Oncol Biol Phys* **65**(1): 91–99.

13. Cawley, E. P. and C. Hoch-Ligeti (1961). "Association of tissue mast cells and skin tumors." *Arch Dermatol* **83**: 92–96.

14. Chaudhuri, A., S. Nielsen, M. L. Elkjaer, V. Zbrzezna, F. Fang and A. O. Pogo (1997). "Detection of Duffy antigen in the plasma membranes and caveolae of vascular endothelial and epithelial cells of nonerythroid organs." *Blood* **89**(2):701–712.

15. Chaudhuri, A., J. Polyakova, V. Zbrzezna, K. Williams, S. Gulati and A. O. Pogo (1993). "Cloning of glycoprotein D cDNA, which encodes the major subunit of the Duffy blood group system and the receptor for the Plasmodium vivax malaria parasite." *Proc Natl Acad Sci U S A* **90**(22): 10793–10797.

16. Colotta, F., F. Re, M. Muzio, R. Bertini, N. Polentarutti, M. Sironi, J. G. Giri, S. K. Dower, J. E. Sims and A. Mantovani (1993). "Interleukin-1 type II receptor: a decoy target for IL-1 that is regulated by IL-4." *Science* **261**(5120): 472–475.

17. Coussens, L. M. and Z. Werb (2002). "Inflammation and cancer." *Nature* **420**(6917): 860–867.

18. Dahut, W. L., J. L. Gulley, P. M. Arlen, Y. Liu, K. M. Fedenko, S. M. Steinberg, J. J. Wright, H. Parnes, C. C. Chen, E. Jones, C. E. Parker, W. M. Linehan and W. D. Figg (2004). "Randomized phase II trial of docetaxel plus thalidomide in androgen-independent prostate cancer." *J Clin Oncol* **22**(13): 2532–2539.

19. Darbonne, W. C., G. C. Rice, M. A. Mohler, T. Apple, C. A. Hebert, A. J. Valente and J. B. Baker (1991). "Red blood cells are a sink for interleukin 8, a leukocyte chemotaxin." *J Clin Invest* **88**(4): 1362–1369.

20. Dawson, T. C., A. B. Lentsch, Z. Wang, J. E. Cowhig, A. Rot, N. Maeda and S. C. Peiper (2000). "Exaggerated response to endotoxin in mice lacking the Duffy antigen/receptor for chemokines (DARC)." *Blood* **96**(5): 1681–1684.

21. De Marzo, A. M., M. J. Putzi and W. G. Nelson (2001). "New concepts in the pathology of prostatic epithelial carcinogenesis." *Urology* **57**(4 Suppl 1): 103–114.

22. Dennis, L. K., C. F. Lynch and J. C. Torner (2002). "Epidemiologic association between prostatitis and prostate cancer." *Urology* **60**(1): 78–83.

23. Drake, C. G., E. Jaffee and D. M. Pardoll (2006). "Mechanisms of immune evasion by tumors." *Adv Immunol* **90**: 51–81.

24. Du, J., J. Luan, H. Liu, T. O. Daniel, S. Peiper, T. S. Chen, Y. Yu, L. W. Horton, L. B. Nanney, R. M. Strieter and A. Richmond (2002). "Potential role for Duffy antigen chemokine-binding protein in angiogenesis and maintenance of homeostasis in response to stress." *J Leukoc Biol* **71**(1): 141–153.

25. Dudley, M. E. and S. A. Rosenberg (2003). "Adoptive-cell-transfer therapy for the treatment of patients with cancer." *Nat Rev Cancer* **3**(9): 666–675.

26. Duncan, L. M., L. A. Richards and M. C. Mihm, Jr. (1998). "Increased mast cell density in invasive melanoma." *J Cutan Pathol* **25**(1): 11–15.

27. Ferrer, F. A., L. J. Miller, R. I. Andrawis, S. H. Kurtzman, P. C. Albertsen, V. P. Laudone and D. L. Kreutzer (1998). "Angiogenesis and prostate cancer: in vivo and in vitro expression of angiogenesis factors by prostate cancer cells." *Urology* **51**(1): 161–167.

28. Figg, W. D., W. Dahut, P. Duray, M. Hamilton, A. Tompkins, S. M. Steinberg, E. Jones, A. Premkumar, W. M. Linehan, M. K. Floeter, C. C. Chen, S. Dixon, D. R. Kohler, E. A. Kruger, E. Gubish, J. M. Pluda and E. Reed (2001)."A randomized phase II trial of thalidomide, an angiogenesis inhibitor, in patients with androgen-independent prostate cancer." *Clin Cancer Res* **7**(7): 1888–1893.

29. Fra, A. M., M. Locati, K. Otero, M. Sironi, P. Signorelli, M. L. Massardi, M. Gobbi, A. Vecchi, S. Sozzani and A. Mantovani (2003)."Cutting edge: scavenging of inflammatory CC chemokines by the promiscuous putatively silent chemokine receptor D6." *J Immunol* **170**(5): 2279–2282.

30. Fulkerson, P. C., N. Zimmermann, L. M. Hassman, F. D. Finkelman and M. E. Rothenberg (2004)."Pulmonary chemokine expression is coordinately regulated by STAT1, STAT6, and IFN-gamma." *J Immunol* **173**(12): 7565–7574.

31. Garcia, M., Jemal A, Ward EM, Center MM, Hao Y, Siegel RL and T. MJ (2007). Global Cancer Facts & Figures 2007. Atlanta, GA, American Cancer Society, 2007.

32. Gasparian, A. V., Y. J. Yao, D. Kowalczyk, L. A. Lyakh, A. Karseladze, T. J. Slaga and I. V. Budunova (2002)."The role of IKK in constitutive activation of NF-kappaB transcription factor in prostate carcinoma cells." *J Cell Sci* **115**(Pt 1): 141–151.

33. Gosling, J., D. J. Dairaghi, Y. Wang, M. Hanley, D. Talbot, Z. Miao and T. J. Schall (2000)."Cutting edge: identification of a novel chemokine receptor that binds dendritic cell- and T cell-active chemokines including ELC, SLC, and TECK." *J Immunol* **164**(6): 2851–2856.

34. Hadley, T. J., Z. H. Lu, K. Wasniowska, A. W. Martin, S. C. Peiper, J. Hesselgesser and R. Horuk (1994)."Postcapillary venule endothelial cells in kidney express a multispecific chemokine receptor that is structurally and functionally identical to the erythroid isoform, which is the Duffy blood group antigen." *J Clin Invest* **94**(3): 985–991.

35. Haverkamp, J., B. Charbonneau and T. L. Ratliff (2007). "Prostate inflammation and its potential impact on prostate cancer: A current review." *J Cell Biochem.*

36. Heidemann, J., H. Ogawa, M. B. Dwinell, P. Rafiee, C. Maaser, H. R. Gockel, M. F. Otterson, D. M. Ota, N. Lugering, W. Domschke and D. G. Binion (2003). "Angiogenic effects of interleukin 8 (CXCL8) in human intestinal microvascular endothelial cells are mediated by CXCR2." *J Biol Chem* **278**(10): 8508–8515.

37. Helbig, G., K. W. Christopherson, 2nd, P. Bhat-Nakshatri, S. Kumar, H. Kishimoto, K. D. Miller, H. E. Broxmeyer and H. Nakshatri (2003)."NF-kappaB promotes breast cancer cell migration and metastasis by inducing the expression of the chemokine receptor CXCR4." *J Biol Chem* **278**(24): 21631–21638.

38. Horton, L. W., Y. Yu, S. Zaja-Milatovic, R. M. Strieter and A. Richmond (2007). "Opposing roles of murine duffy antigen receptor for chemokine and murine CXC chemokine receptor-2 receptors in murine melanoma tumor growth." *Cancer Res* **67**(20): 9791–9799.

39. Horuk, R., C. E. Chitnis, W. C. Darbonne, T. J. Colby, A. Rybicki, T. J. Hadley and L. H. Miller (1993)."A receptor for the malarial parasite Plasmodium vivax: the erythrocyte chemokine receptor." *Science* **261**(5125): 1182–1184.

40. Huang, J., J. L. Yao, L. Zhang, P. A. Bourne, A. M. Quinn, P. A. di Sant'Agnese and J. E. Reeder (2005)."Differential expression of interleukin-8 and its receptors in the neuroendocrine and non-neuroendocrine compartments of prostate cancer." *Am J Pathol* **166**(6): 1807–1815.

41. Hub, E. and A. Rot (1998)."Binding of RANTES, MCP-1, MCP-3, and MIP-1alpha to cells in human skin." *Am J Pathol* **152**(3): 749–757.

42. Inoue, K., J. W. Slaton, B. Y. Eve, S. J. Kim, P. Perrotte, M. D. Balbay, S. Yano, M. Bar-Eli, R. Radinsky, C. A. Pettaway and C. P. Dinney (2000)."Interleukin 8 expression regulates tumorigenicity and metastases in androgen-independent prostate cancer." *Clin Cancer Res* **6**(5): 2104–2119.

43. Jamieson, T., D. N. Cook, R. J. Nibbs, A. Rot, C. Nixon, P. McLean, A. Alcami, S. A. Lira, M. Wiekowski and G. J. Graham (2005). "The chemokine receptor D6 limits the inflammatory response in vivo." *Nat Immunol* **6**(4): 403–411.
44. Kiessling, A., S. Fussel, R. Wehner, M. Bachmann, M. P. Wirth, E. P. Rieber and M. Schmitz (2007). "Advances in Specific Immunotherapy for Prostate Cancer." *Eur Urol* **53**(4): 694–708.
45. Kim, S. J., H. Uehara, T. Karashima, M. McCarty, N. Shih and I. J. Fidler (2001). "Expression of interleukin-8 correlates with angiogenesis, tumorigenicity, and metastasis of human prostate cancer cells implanted orthotopically in nude mice." *Neoplasia* **3**(1): 33–42.
46. Konig, J. E., T. Senge, E. P. Allhoff and W. Konig (2004). "Analysis of the inflammatory network in benign prostate hyperplasia and prostate cancer." *Prostate* **58**(2): 121–129.
47. Lee, J. S., C. W. Frevert, M. M. Wurfel, S. C. Peiper, V. A. Wong, K. K. Ballman, J. T. Ruzinski, J. S. Rhim, T. R. Martin and R. B. Goodman (2003). "Duffy antigen facilitates movement of chemokine across the endothelium in vitro and promotes neutrophil transmigration in vitro and in vivo." *J Immunol* **170**(10): 5244–5251.
48. Lehrer, S., E. J. Diamond, B. Mamkine, N. N. Stone and R. G. Stock (2004). "Serum interleukin-8 is elevated in men with prostate cancer and bone metastases." *Technol Cancer Res Treat* **3**(5): 411.
49. Liotta, L. A., J. Kleinerman and G. M. Saidel (1974). "Quantitative relationships of intravascular tumor cells, tumor vessels, and pulmonary metastases following tumor implantation." *Cancer Res* **34**(5): 997–1004.
50. Liotta, L. A., M. G. Saidel and J. Kleinerman (1976). "The significance of hematogenous tumor cell clumps in the metastatic process." *Cancer Res* **36**(3): 889–894.
51. Loberg, R. D., C. Ying, M. Craig, L. Yan, L. A. Snyder and K. J. Pienta (2007). "CCL2 as an important mediator of prostate cancer growth in vivo through the regulation of macrophage infiltration." *Neoplasia* **9**(7): 556–562.
52. Lu, Y., Z. Cai, D. L. Galson, G. Xiao, Y. Liu, D. E. George, M. F. Melhem, Z. Yao and J. Zhang (2006). "Monocyte chemotactic protein-1 (MCP-1) acts as a paracrine and autocrine factor for prostate cancer growth and invasion." *Prostate* **66**(12): 1311–1318.
53. Luo, H., A. Chaudhuri, V. Zbrzezna, Y. He and A. O. Pogo (2000). "Deletion of the murine Duffy gene (Dfy) reveals that the Duffy receptor is functionally redundant." *Mol Cell Biol* **20**(9): 3097–3101.
54. Mantovani, A. (1999). "The chemokine system: redundancy for robust outputs." *Immunol Today* **20**(6): 254–257.
55. Mantovani, A., M. Locati, A. Vecchi, S. Sozzani and P. Allavena (2001). "Decoy receptors: a strategy to regulate inflammatory cytokines and chemokines." *Trends Immunol* **22**(6): 328–336.
56. Martinez de la Torre, Y., C. Buracchi, E. M. Borroni, J. Dupor, R. Bonecchi, M. Nebuloni, F. Pasqualini, A. Doni, E. Lauri, C. Agostinis, R. Bulla, D. N. Cook, B. Haribabu, P. Meroni, D. Rukavina, L. Vago, F. Tedesco, A. Vecchi, S. A. Lira, M. Locati and A. Mantovani (2007). "Protection against inflammation- and autoantibody-caused fetal loss by the chemokine decoy receptor D6." *Proc Natl Acad Sci U S A* **104**(7): 2319–2324.
57. Martinez de la Torre, Y., M. Locati, C. Buracchi, J. Dupor, D. N. Cook, R. Bonecchi, M. Nebuloni, D. Rukavina, L. Vago, A. Vecchi, S. A. Lira and A. Mantovani (2005). "Increased inflammation in mice deficient for the chemokine decoy receptor D6." *Eur J Immunol* **35**(5): 1342–1346.
58. Maxwell, P. J., R. Gallagher, A. Seaton, C. Wilson, P. Scullin, J. Pettigrew, I. J. Stratford, K. J. Williams, P. G. Johnston and D. J. Waugh (2007). "HIF-1 and NF-kappaB-mediated upregulation of CXCR1 and CXCR2 expression promotes cell survival in hypoxic prostate cancer cells." *Oncogene* **26**(52): 7333–7345.
59. Miller, L. H., S. J. Mason, D. F. Clyde and M. H. McGinniss (1976). "The resistance factor to Plasmodium vivax in blacks. The Duffy-blood-group genotype, FyFy." *N Engl J Med* **295**(6): 302–304.

60. Miller, L. H., S. J. Mason, J. A. Dvorak, M. H. McGinniss and I. K. Rothman (1975). "Erythrocyte receptors for (Plasmodium knowlesi) malaria: Duffy blood group determinants." *Science* **189**(4202): 561–563.
61. Mochizuki, H., A. Matsubara, J. Teishima, K. Mutaguchi, H. Yasumoto, R. Dahiya, T. Usui and K. Kamiya (2004). "Interaction of ligand-receptor system between stromal-cell-derived factor-1 and CXC chemokine receptor 4 in human prostate cancer: a possible predictor of metastasis." *Biochem Biophys Res Commun* **320**(3): 656–663.
62. Moore, B. B., D. A. Arenberg, K. Stoy, T. Morgan, C. L. Addison, S. B. Morris, M. Glass, C. Wilke, Y. Y. Xue, S. Sitterding, S. L. Kunkel, M. D. Burdick and R. M. Strieter (1999). "Distinct CXC chemokines mediate tumorigenicity of prostate cancer cells." *Am J Pathol* **154**(5): 1503–1512.
63. Movsas, B., J. D. Chapman, E. M. Horwitz, W. H. Pinover, R. E. Greenberg, A. L. Hanlon, R. Iyer and G. E. Hanks (1999). "Hypoxic regions exist in human prostate carcinoma." *Urology* **53**(1): 11–18.
64. Murphy, C., M. McGurk, J. Pettigrew, A. Santinelli, R. Mazzucchelli, P. G. Johnston, R. Montironi and D. J. Waugh (2005). "Nonapical and cytoplasmic expression of interleukin-8, CXCR1, and CXCR2 correlates with cell proliferation and microvessel density in prostate cancer." *Clin Cancer Res* **11**(11): 4117–4127.
65. Murphy, P. M. (1994). "The molecular biology of leukocyte chemoattractant receptors." *Annu Rev Immunol* **12**: 593–633.
66. Nagpal, M. L., J. Davis and T. Lin (2006). "Overexpression of CXCL10 in human prostate LNCaP cells activates its receptor (CXCR3) expression and inhibits cell proliferation." *Biochim Biophys Acta* **1762**(9): 811–818.
67. Nelson, W. G., A. M. De Marzo and W. B. Isaacs (2003). "Prostate cancer." *N Engl J Med* **349**(4): 366–381.
68. Nelson, W. G., T. L. DeWeese and A. M. DeMarzo (2002). "The diet, prostate inflammation, and the development of prostate cancer." *Cancer Metastasis Rev* **21**(1): 3–16.
69. Neote, K., W. Darbonne, J. Ogez, R. Horuk and T. J. Schall (1993). "Identification of a promiscuous inflammatory peptide receptor on the surface of red blood cells." *J Biol Chem* **268**(17): 12247–12249.
70. Neote, K., J. Y. Mak, L. F. Kolakowski, Jr. and T. J. Schall (1994). "Functional and biochemical analysis of the cloned Duffy antigen: identity with the red blood cell chemokine receptor." *Blood* **84**(1): 44–52.
71. Nibbs, R., G. Graham and A. Rot (2003). "Chemokines on the move: control by the chemokine "interceptors" Duffy blood group antigen and D6." *Semin Immunol* **15**(5): 287–294.
72. Nibbs, R. J., D. S. Gilchrist, V. King, A. Ferra, S. Forrow, K. D. Hunter and G. J. Graham (2007). "The atypical chemokine receptor D6 suppresses the development of chemically induced skin tumors." *J Clin Invest* **117**(7): 1884–1892.
73. Nibbs, R. J., S. M. Wylie, J. Yang, N. R. Landau and G. J. Graham (1997). "Cloning and characterization of a novel promiscuous human beta-chemokine receptor D6." *J Biol Chem* **272**(51): 32078–32083.
74. Palayoor, S. T., M. Y. Youmell, S. K. Calderwood, C. N. Coleman and B. D. Price (1999). "Constitutive activation of IkappaB kinase alpha and NF-kappaB in prostate cancer cells is inhibited by ibuprofen." *Oncogene* **18**(51): 7389–7394.
75. Peiper, S. C., Z. X. Wang, K. Neote, A. W. Martin, H. J. Showell, M. J. Conklyn, K. Ogborne, T. J. Hadley, Z. H. Lu, J. Hesselgesser and R. Horuk (1995). "The Duffy antigen/receptor for chemokines (DARC) is expressed in endothelial cells of Duffy negative individuals who lack the erythrocyte receptor." *J Exp Med* **181**(4): 1311–1317.
76. Pirtskhalaishvili, G. and J. B. Nelson (2000). "Endothelium-derived factors as paracrine mediators of prostate cancer progression." *Prostate* **44**(1): 77–87.
77. Ponomaryov, T., A. Peled, I. Petit, R. S. Taichman, L. Habler, J. Sandbank, F. Arenzana-Seisdedos, A. Magerus, A. Caruz, N. Fujii, A. Nagler, M. Lahav, M. Szyper-Kravitz,

D. Zipori and T. Lapidot (2000)."Induction of the chemokine stromal-derived factor-1 following DNA damage improves human stem cell function." *J Clin Invest* **106**(11): 1331–1339.

78. Putzi, M. J. and A. M. De Marzo (2000)."Morphologic transitions between proliferative inflammatory atrophy and high-grade prostatic intraepithelial neoplasia." *Urology* **56**(5): 828–832.

79. Quinn, M. and P. Babb (2002a)."Patterns and trends in prostate cancer incidence, survival, prevalence and mortality. Part I: international comparisons." *BJU Int* **90**(2): 162–173.

80. Quinn, M. and P. Babb (2002b)."Patterns and trends in prostate cancer incidence, survival, prevalence and mortality. Part II: individual countries." *BJU Int* **90**(2): 174–184.

81. Rabinovich, G. A., D. Gabrilovich and E. M. Sotomayor (2007)."Immunosuppressive strategies that are mediated by tumor cells." *Annu Rev Immunol* **25**: 267–296.

82. Reiland, J., L. T. Furcht and J. B. McCarthy (1999)."CXC-chemokines stimulate invasion and chemotaxis in prostate carcinoma cells through the CXCR2 receptor." *Prostate* **41**(2): 78–88.

83. Rollins, B. J. (1997)."Chemokines." *Blood* **90**(3): 909–928.

84. Romero, S., G. Stanton, J. DeFelice, F. Schreiber, R. Rago and M. Fishman (2007). "Phase II trial of thalidomide and daily oral dexamethasone for treatment of hormone refractory prostate cancer progressing after chemotherapy." *Urol Oncol* **25**(4): 284–290.

85. Rosenberg, S. A. (1997)."Cancer vaccines based on the identification of genes encoding cancer regression antigens." *Immunol Today* **18**(4): 175–182.

86. Ross, J. S., K. E. Gray, I. J. Webb, G. S. Gray, M. Rolfe, D. P. Schenkein, D. M. Nanus, M. I. Millowsky and N. H. Bander (2005)."Antibody-based therapeutics: focus on prostate cancer." *Cancer Metastasis Rev* **24**(4): 521–537.

87. Rot, A. (2003)."In situ binding assay for studying chemokine interactions with endothelial cells." *J Immunol Methods* **273**(1–2): 63–71.

88. Sato, E., S. H. Olson, J. Ahn, B. Bundy, H. Nishikawa, F. Qian, A. A. Jungbluth, D. Frosina, S. Gnjatic, C. Ambrosone, J. Kepner, T. Odunsi, G. Ritter, S. Lele, Y. T. Chen, H. Ohtani, L. J. Old and K. Odunsi (2005)."Intraepithelial CD8 + tumor-infiltrating lymphocytes and a high CD8 + /regulatory T cell ratio are associated with favorable prognosis in ovarian cancer." *Proc Natl Acad Sci U S A* **102**(51): 18538–18543.

89. Shankaran, V., H. Ikeda, A. T. Bruce, J. M. White, P. E. Swanson, L. J. Old and R. D. Schreiber (2001)."IFNgamma and lymphocytes prevent primary tumour development and shape tumour immunogenicity." *Nature* **410**(6832): 1107–1111.

90. Shen, H. and A. B. Lentsch (2004)."Progressive dysregulation of transcription factors NF-kappa B and STAT1 in prostate cancer cells causes proangiogenic production of CXC chemokines." *Am J Physiol Cell Physiol* **286**(4): C840–847.

91. Shen, H., R. Schuster, B. Lu, S. E. Waltz and A. B. Lentsch (2006)."Critical and opposing roles of the chemokine receptors CXCR2 and CXCR3 in prostate tumor growth." *Prostate* **66**(16): 1721–1728.

92. Shen, H., R. Schuster, K. F. Stringer, S. E. Waltz and A. B. Lentsch (2006)."The Duffy antigen/receptor for chemokines (DARC) regulates prostate tumor growth." *FASEB J* **20**(1): 59–64.

93. Sierro, F., C. Biben, L. Martinez-Munoz, M. Mellado, R. M. Ransohoff, M. Li, B. Woehl, H. Leung, J. Groom, M. Batten, R. P. Harvey, A. C. Martinez, C. R. Mackay and F. Mackay (2007)."Disrupted cardiac development but normal hematopoiesis in mice deficient in the second CXCL12/SDF-1 receptor, CXCR7." *Proc Natl Acad Sci U S A* **104**(37): 14759–14764.

94. Strieter, R. M., P. J. Polverini, S. L. Kunkel, D. A. Arenberg, M. D. Burdick, J. Kasper, J. Dzuiba, J. Van Damme, A. Walz, D. Marriott and et al. (1995)."The functional role of the ELR motif in CXC chemokine-mediated angiogenesis." *J Biol Chem* **270**(45): 27348–27357.

95. Suh, J., F. Payvandi, L. C. Edelstein, P. S. Amenta, W. X. Zong, C. Gelinas and A. B. Rabson (2002)."Mechanisms of constitutive NF-kappaB activation in human prostate cancer cells." *Prostate* **52**(3): 183–200.

96. Sun, Y. X., M. Fang, J. Wang, C. R. Cooper, K. J. Pienta and R. S. Taichman (2007). "Expression and activation of alpha v beta 3 integrins by SDF-1/CXC12 increases the aggressiveness of prostate cancer cells." *Prostate* **67**(1): 61–73.

97. Sun, Y. X., A. Schneider, Y. Jung, J. Wang, J. Dai, K. Cook, N. I. Osman, A. J. Koh-Paige, H. Shim, K. J. Pienta, E. T. Keller, L. K. McCauley and R. S. Taichman (2005)."Skeletal localization and neutralization of the SDF-1(CXCL12)/CXCR4 axis blocks prostate cancer metastasis and growth in osseous sites in vivo." *J Bone Miner Res* **20**(2): 318–329.

98. Sun, Y. X., J. Wang, C. E. Shelburne, D. E. Lopatin, A. M. Chinnaiyan, M. A. Rubin, K. J. Pienta and R. S. Taichman (2003)."Expression of CXCR4 and CXCL12 (SDF-1) in human prostate cancers (PCa) in vivo." *J Cell Biochem* **89**(3): 462–473.

99. Taichman, R. S., C. Cooper, E. T. Keller, K. J. Pienta, N. S. Taichman and L. K. McCauley (2002)."Use of the stromal cell-derived factor-1/CXCR4 pathway in prostate cancer metastasis to bone." *Cancer Res* **62**(6): 1832–1837.

100. Uehara, H., P. Troncoso, D. Johnston, C. D. Bucana, C. Dinney, Z. Dong, I. J. Fidler and C. A. Pettaway (2005)."Expression of interleukin-8 gene in radical prostatectomy specimens is associated with advanced pathologic stage." *Prostate* **64**(1): 40–49.

101. Veltri, R. W., M. C. Miller, G. Zhao, A. Ng, G. M. Marley, G. L. Wright, Jr., R. L. Vessella and D. Ralph (1999)."Interleukin-8 serum levels in patients with benign prostatic hyperplasia and prostate cancer." *Urology* **53**(1): 139–147.

102. Wang, J., J. Dai, Y. Jung, C. L. Wei, Y. Wang, A. M. Havens, P. J. Hogg, E. T. Keller, K. J. Pienta, J. E. Nor, C. Y. Wang and R. S. Taichman (2007)."A glycolytic mechanism regulating an angiogenic switch in prostate cancer." *Cancer Res* **67**(1): 149–159.

103. Wang, J., Y. Shiozawa, J. Wang, Y. Wang, Y. Jung, K. J. Pienta, R. Mehra, R. Loberg and R. S. Taichmann (2007)."The Role of CXCR7/RDC1 as a Chemokine Receptor for CXCL12/SDF-1 in Prostate Cancer." *J Biol Chem* **283**(7): 4283–4294.

104. Wang, R. F. (2001)."The role of MHC class II-restricted tumor antigens and CD4 + T cells in antitumor immunity." *Trends Immunol* **22**(5): 269–276.

105. Weber, M., E. Blair, C. V. Simpson, M. O'Hara, P. E. Blackburn, A. Rot, G. J. Graham and R. J. Nibbs (2004)."The chemokine receptor D6 constitutively traffics to and from the cell surface to internalize and degrade chemokines." *Mol Biol Cell* **15**(5): 2492–2508.

106. Weidner, N., P. R. Carroll, J. Flax, W. Blumenfeld and J. Folkman (1993)."Tumor angiogenesis correlates with metastasis in invasive prostate carcinoma." *Am J Pathol* **143**(2): 401–409.

107. Whitehead, G. S., T. Wang, L. M. DeGraff, J. W. Card, S. A. Lira, G. J. Graham and D. N. Cook (2007)."The chemokine receptor D6 has opposing effects on allergic inflammation and airway reactivity." *Am J Respir Crit Care Med* **175**(3): 243–249.

108. Zlotnik, A. and O. Yoshie (2000)."Chemokines: a new classification system and their role in immunity." *Immunity* **12**(2): 121–127.

Index

Printed in the United States
147238LV00003B/90/P